# KETO
# SNACKS

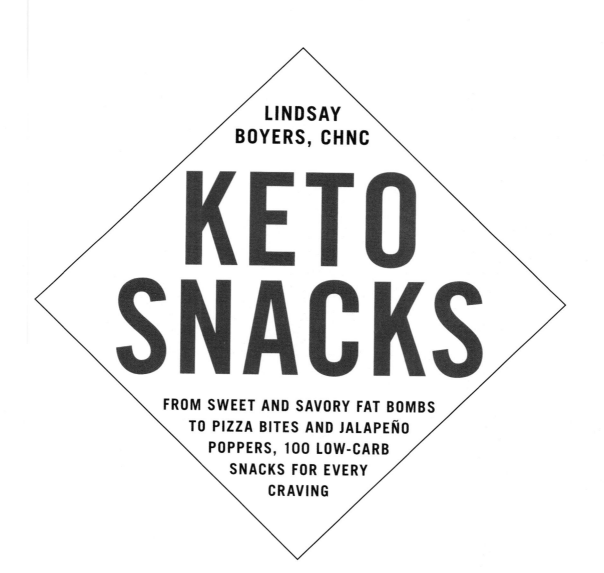

LINDSAY
BOYERS, CHNC

# KETO SNACKS

FROM SWEET AND SAVORY FAT BOMBS
TO PIZZA BITES AND JALAPEÑO
POPPERS, 100 LOW-CARB
SNACKS FOR EVERY
CRAVING

**ADAMS MEDIA**

NEW YORK  LONDON  TORONTO  SYDNEY  NEW DELHI

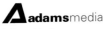

Adams Media
An Imprint of Simon & Schuster, Inc.
57 Littlefield Street
Avon, Massachusetts 02322

First Adams Media trade paperback edition November 2018

ADAMS MEDIA and colophon are trademarks of Simon & Schuster.

For information about special discounts for bulk purchases, please contact Simon & Schuster Special Sales at 1-866-506-1949 or business@simonandschuster.com.

The Simon & Schuster Speakers Bureau can bring authors to your live event. For more information or to book an event contact the Simon & Schuster Speakers Bureau at 1-866-248-3049 or visit our website at www.simonspeakers.com.

Interior design by Sylvia McArdle
Photographs by James Stefiuk
Nutritional statistics by Melinda Boyd

Manufactured in the United States of America

10   9   8   7   6   5   4   3   2   1

Library of Congress Cataloging-in-Publication Data
Boyers, Lindsay, author.
Keto snacks / Lindsay Boyers, CHNC.
Avon, Massachusetts: Adams Media, 2018.
Includes index.
LCCN 2018023276 | ISBN 9781507209202 (pb) | ISBN 9781507209219 (ebook)
Subjects: LCSH: Ketogenic diet--Recipes. | Reducing diets--Recipes. | Low-carbohydrate diet--Recipes. | BISAC: COOKING / Health & Healing / Low Carbohydrate. | COOKING / Methods / Quick & Easy. | HEALTH & FITNESS / Diets.
Classification: LCC RM222.2 .B64827 2018 | DDC 641.5/6383--dc23
LC record available at https://lccn.loc.gov/2018023276

ISBN 978-1-5072-0920-2
ISBN 978-1-5072-0921-9 (ebook)

Contains material adapted from the following title published by Adams Media, an Imprint of Simon & Schuster, Inc.: *The Everything® Ketogenic Diet Cookbook* by Lindsay Boyers, CHNC, copyright © 2017, ISBN 978-1-5072-0626-3.

*To my mom, Lola. Thank you for guiding me, yet allowing me to make my own decisions. Thank you for supporting me, yet never pushing me. Thank you for honoring my strange requests and only buying me pens for Christmas one year. You helped pave the way for my writing career and I couldn't appreciate you more. I love you.*

# CONTENTS

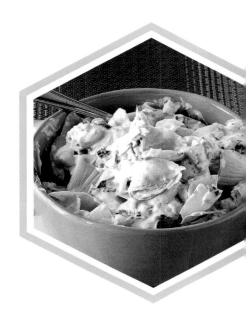

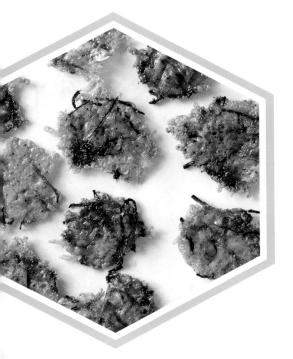

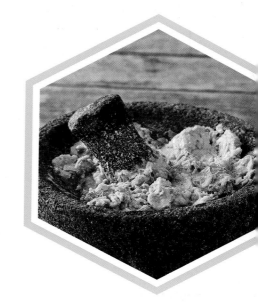

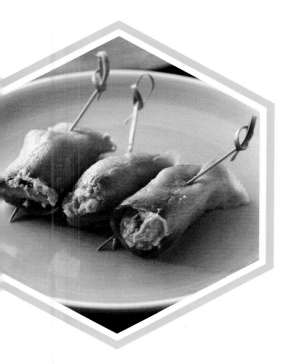

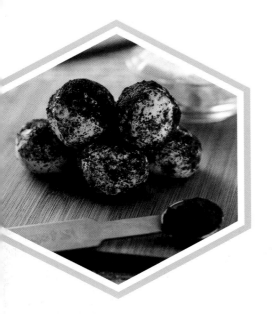

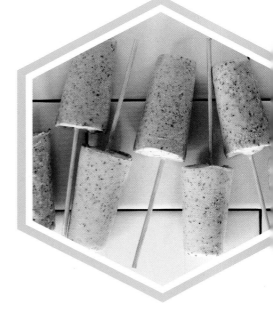

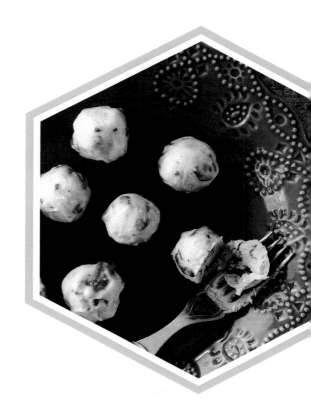

# INTRODUCTION

*Pumpkin Pie Coconut Crisps*

*Bacon Jalapeño Balls*

*Hazelnut Truffles*

*Cheesy Muffin Prosciutto Cup*

Who doesn't love a snack? Snacks are not only delicious; they are essential to making sure you are getting the proper amounts of nutrients in your day. Unfortunately, most snack foods are high in sugar, salt, trans fats, artificial ingredients, or all of the above. But with *Keto Snacks* you'll find snacks that not only calm your cravings but also fit into your healthy lifestyle. Now you can snack and lose weight too!

Inside you'll find 100 keto-approved snacks to satisfy your hunger and keep you on track. You'll also find easy tips on how to incorporate snacking into your daily routine *without* going overboard.

The key to snacking on the ketogenic diet is to snack smartly. You can do this by making sure your snacks are healthy and appropriate for your meal plan, and the best way to do that is to make them yourself. That way, you can control what goes into them—no artificial ingredients here!

You'll also be able to control macronutrients and determine which snacks are best for you on any given day. Need more fat? Have a fat bomb. Looking to balance out your protein needs? Choose some Deli Rollups—whatever you need, *Keto Snacks* has you covered.

Choosing the right types of snacks and following these simple tips can make snacking an integral part of your success on a ketogenic diet. When you snack smartly and mindfully, you'll be on your way to becoming a better, healthier you!

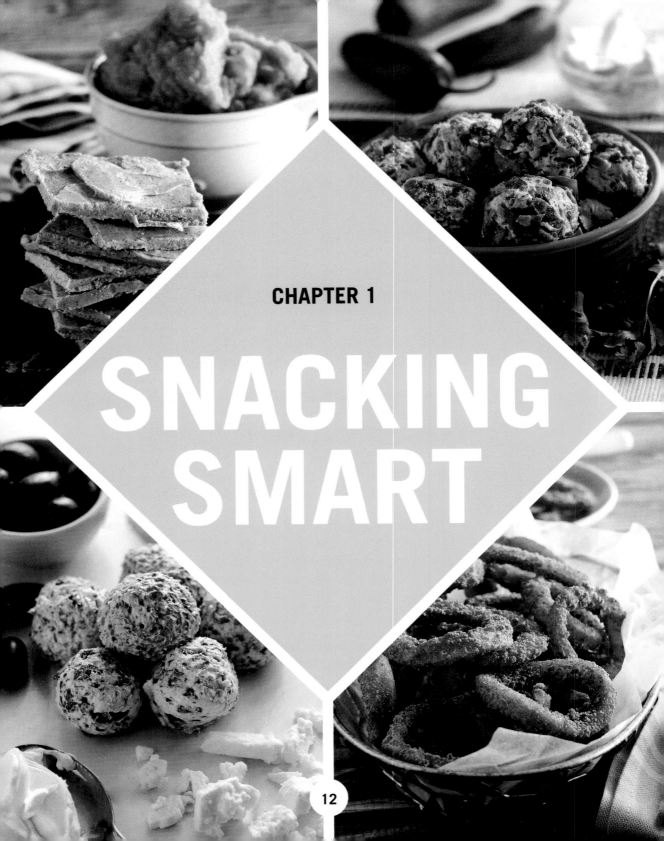

CHAPTER 1

# SNACKING SMART

The ketogenic diet is designed to keep your blood sugar levels steady and your hunger at bay, but even then there will be times when you'll just want or need a snack—and there's nothing wrong with that! Sometimes snacking gets a bad rap, but it's not snacking itself that's usually the problem; it's the types of food people choose and amounts they eat. When you choose healthy snacks on the ketogenic diet and make sure not to overdo it on your portions, they can be a beneficial part of your plan.

# WHAT IS THE KETOGENIC DIET?

The ketogenic diet, lovingly nicknamed "keto," is a high-fat, very low-carbohydrate diet that allows moderate amounts of protein. Although keto shares similar characteristics with popular low-carb diets like Atkins, it's different because the intent is to induce ketosis, which may or may not happen on your typical low-carbohydrate diet.

## Explaining Ketosis

Your body's preferred energy source is carbohydrates. When you eat carbohydrates, your body breaks them down into the simple sugar glucose, which travels into your bloodstream where it's picked up by insulin. Insulin either carries the glucose into your cells for immediate use, or the glucose is converted to glycogen and then stored in your liver to be used for energy at a later time, like in between meals. As long

### Fat versus Carbohydrates

One of the benefits of using fat for energy instead of carbohydrates is that your body can only store a certain amount of carbohydrates, but its ability to store fat is endless. That means that if you rely on carbohydrates for energy, you'll eventually reach a point at which that energy runs out because stored carbohydrates have also run out.

as you're consistently eating carbohydrates, this cycle will continue. Your body will use the glucose it needs for immediate energy and then store the rest. When you are using carbohydrates for energy, fat is stored in your fat cells and left there indefinitely.

The goal of the ketogenic diet is to restrict carbohydrate intake and interfere with this glucose mechanism. In the absence of carbohydrates, your body will turn to fat—its second preferred source—for energy.

To convert fat into usable energy, the liver breaks it down into fatty acids and then breaks down these fatty acids into energy-rich substances called ketones or ketone bodies. The presence of ketone bodies in the blood is called ketosis. When there are ketones in your blood and you've entered a state of ketosis, it indicates that your body is burning fat for energy instead of carbohydrates.

The exact percentage of each macronutrient you need to kick your body into ketosis is different from person to person, but in general the macronutrient ratio for a ketogenic diet falls into the following ranges:

- 60–75 percent of calories from fat
- 15–30 percent of calories from protein
- 5–10 percent of calories from carbohydrates

When following a ketogenic diet, it's likely that you'll have to play around with these numbers a little bit to determine which macronutrient ratios are right for you. Once you've figured them out, you can design your meals and snacks around them. You can verify that you're in ketosis by using test strips called ketone strips, which are available at most local drugstores. There are also symptoms that tend to occur in the very beginning stages of ketosis that signal your success.

## How Ketone Strips Work

Ketone strips work by measuring the amount of acetoacetate—one of the two main ketone bodies—in your urine. To use a ketone strip, you'll need to collect a urine sample in a clean container, hold the stick in the urine, and then wait fifteen seconds. The strip will change color, and you can compare it to a color chart included with the test strips. It's important to note, however, that ketone strips are not entirely accurate because urine strips only measure the amount of ketones expelled from your body, not the actual amount in your blood.

### Signs That You Are in Ketosis

Once you've entered ketosis, you may experience some physical symptoms. In many cases, these symptoms begin within one week of starting a strict ketogenic diet. For other people, it can take a bit longer—up to three months. When physical symptoms do develop, they are pretty similar for everyone. The most common signs of ketosis include:

- Bad breath
- Decreased appetite and nausea
- Cold hands and feet
- Increased urinary frequency

- Difficulty sleeping
- Metallic taste in the mouth
- Dry mouth
- Increased thirst

As your body adjusts to using fat for fuel instead of carbohydrates, the unpleasant physical symptoms dissipate, and you'll begin to experience the positive benefits of ketosis, which include:

- Increased energy
- Improved mental focus and clarity
- Weight loss

## The Keto "Flu"

When you restrict carbohydrates, your hormones and electrolytes go through changes as they work to become balanced. As these changes occur, you may experience some uncomfortable symptoms, such as fatigue, headaches, nausea, cramps, diarrhea, brain fog, and upset stomach. Because these symptoms closely resemble those of the flu,

### A Note on Sports Drinks

Sports drinks are known for their high electrolyte content, but they're also full of sugar and artificial ingredients. The lower-sugar versions contain artificial sweeteners in place of sugar, and while technically the macronutrients may fall into your ketogenic diet, they're not good for you for other reasons. Try to stay away from these types of artificial drinks and opt for natural sources of electrolytes.

this stage of adapting to ketosis is referred to as the "keto flu." The duration of symptoms varies from person to person, but in most cases keto flu goes away in two days to one week. To reduce the severity of keto flu symptoms, stay hydrated by drinking filtered water and electrolyte-rich fluids like bone broth and pickle juice.

## WHY YOU SHOULD SNACK

While the ketogenic diet is designed to keep your blood sugar levels stable, strategic snacking can help keep your hunger in check. Eating well-balanced, healthy snacks can also help you meet your macronutrient and micronutrient needs for the day. You can design your meal plan to include one or two snacks per day, but be careful not to overdo it. Because ketogenic snacks are high in fat, they're also naturally high in calories.

In addition to helping meet your dietary needs, snacking can also help curb your appetite and prevent you from overeating at meals or reaching for something unhealthy because you're ravenous and your willpower isn't strong. There's also some evidence that snacking can help lower cholesterol, triglycerides, and LDL—or "bad" cholesterol. Of course, the types of snacks you eat have a major impact on the benefits you'll see, so it's important to snack smartly.

## HOW TO SNACK SMARTLY

Snacking gets a bad rap, but it's not the snacking itself that's usually detrimental; it's a combination of snack choices and bad snacking practices. As with any other diet plan, you want to be smart when it comes to snacking on the ketogenic diet. Eating too much and too often may throw off your macronutrient ratios and could contribute excess calories—preventing weight loss or contributing to weight gain. If weight loss is your goal, you want to be extra mindful of how many snacks you're consuming and when, but incorporating a couple of snacks each day can help keep you on track, especially in the beginning stages when your body is starting to adjust and you're trying to get into the groove of a new way of life.

## Snack Mindfully

One of the biggest downfalls when it comes to snacking is eating too much because you're distracted. It's common for people to snack while they're doing something else, such as watching television or scrolling through their phones, but when you're distracted, it's easier to lose track of how much you're eating. That's because you're not really paying attention, and you're missing the signals that you've had enough. In fact, one study found that people who snacked while highly distracted—in this case, playing a computer game—consumed 69 percent more snacks than other participants who ate without distraction.

To keep your snacking in check, turn the television off and put away your phone. Treat a snack like a meal. Put your food on a plate or in a bowl, sit down to eat it, and savor each bite. Pay attention to the taste and texture. Chew carefully. In addition to helping prevent overeating and binge eating, eating mindfully has been shown to improve digestion and overall food satisfaction and to reduce anxious and negative thoughts about food and your body.

## Prepare Portions

Of course, snacking in front of the television can sometimes be one of the simple pleasures in life, so while it's best not to snack while you're distracted, it's not realistic to think that you'll avoid it forever. If you do snack in front of the television, there are simple snacking "rules" you can follow to make it easier to snack smartly.

Instead of eating out of a large container that has more food in it than you want to eat, portion your snacks out prior to sitting down. For example, if you just made a bunch of Snickerdoodle Roasted Nuts (Chapter 3), put a handful in a little bowl and put the rest away instead of bringing the entire tray to the couch with you. If you have a fresh batch of Maple Nut Bars (Chapter 3), put one on a plate to take with you into the living room and put the rest away for later. This has a double advantage because you won't overeat in the moment, and you'll be happy that you have some healthy keto snacks left over and ready to go the next time you want to reach for a snack.

The same advice can be applied to all snacking, even if you're not in front of the television. Portioning snacks out in advance won't just keep you within your calorie needs; it also makes life a little easier for you when you're on the go. If you always have a preportioned snack ready to go in a bag or airtight container, you can grab it on your way out the door and be ready anytime hunger strikes without having to think about it or scramble at the last minute to try to find a snack.

## Eat Slowly

Just like with your meals, it can take your stomach some time (up to twenty minutes) to register that you're full after a snack. If you eat really quickly, you're more likely to consume more than you need because your stomach won't have adequate time to tell your brain you're full. Eat your snacks slowly and give your stomach a chance to fill up before reaching for more. If after twenty minutes you're still genuinely hungry, have a little more or consider that it might be time for a meal. If you're not actually hungry, but you just want more for the sake of eating or because of boredom, skip it and occupy your mind with something else.

## Work Around Your Meals

While snacking can keep you satiated between meals, your meals should be the star of the show—and they should keep you full for two to three hours. It's normal to eat a couple of snacks during the day, but if you're constantly feeling hungry or reaching for a snack, take a look at your meals and make sure you're getting enough fat. If your meals are balanced and you still find yourself reaching for snacks constantly, try to determine whether you're actually hungry or just bored. If it's the latter, occupy your time with things you enjoy doing to take your mind off food. Go for a walk or write in your journal. Do some yoga or some stretching. Call a friend. (Yes, call and have a conversation instead of texting.) When you busy yourself with other things, you're less likely to eat out of boredom.

## Time Your Snacks

There are no rules about food timing when following a basic keto-genic diet, but timing your snacks can have beneficial effects on both your waistline and your energy levels. Eating a snack two hours after a meal—and two hours before your next meal—can help keep you full and prevent you from reaching for something that's not on your diet plan. It's also helpful to figure out a cutoff time at night when you'll stop eating and give your digestive system time to shut down and do some maintenance.

### Giving Your Digestive System a Rest

According to Satchidananda Panda, a professor at the Salk Institute for Biological Studies and an expert in the fields of biology and circadian rhythms, giving your body an eight- to twelve-hour window without food can help you lose weight, decrease your risk of diabetes and obesity, and lower cholesterol levels. You can incorporate Panda's research into your ketogenic diet plan by having your last snack at eight p.m. and waiting until eight a.m. to eat breakfast—a dietary concept known as intermittent fasting.

# SNACKING AND INTERMITTENT FASTING

Intermittent fasting has become a popular complement to the ketogenic diet. If you're incorporating intermittent fasting into your ketogenic diet plan, you can still snack strategically. You'll just have to time your snacks and make sure they fall into your feeding window.

## What Is Intermittent Fasting?

Intermittent fasting isn't a specific diet; it's a food-timing strategy. It involves alternating set periods of time when you eat with set periods of time when you don't. The period of time when you eat is called your feeding window, and the period of time when you fast is referred to as the fasting window.

For example, someone who is incorporating intermittent fasting into his or her ketogenic diet may decide to eat between the hours of eleven a.m. and seven p.m. and then fast—or consume only water, broth, or coffee—between the hours of seven p.m. and eleven a.m. The idea behind intermittent fasting is that giving your body that rest period between meals allows your digestive system to reset and clean itself. As a result, you lose weight, gain more energy, and experience more mental clarity.

## Timing Your Snacks

You can successfully incorporate snacks into your intermittent fasting plan by timing your snacks during your feeding window. For example, if you're on the eleven a.m. to seven p.m. plan, you could eat breakfast at eleven a.m., eat a snack at one p.m., eat lunch at three p.m., eat another small snack at five p.m., and then finish off with dinner around six-thirty p.m.

# FAT BOMBS VERSUS OTHER KETO SNACKS

Fat bombs fall into the category of keto snacks, but they're a very specific type of snack with a targeted purpose. A standard fat bomb contains about 90 percent fat and very minimal amounts of both carbohydrates and protein. Typically, the two most common ingredients in fat bombs are coconut oil and high-fat dairy products (for those who can tolerate dairy). The purpose of a fat bomb is to give your body an extra dose of fat to use as fuel in between meals or when your daily macronutrient ratio is off and you need a few extra grams of fat to meet your needs so your body remains in ketosis. Fat bombs are also commonly used to satisfy a sweet craving because many of them are made with cocoa or cacao powder, although fat bombs can be savory too. Due to the high fat content of fat bombs, they're naturally high in calories, so eat them mindfully and don't overdo it. Fat bombs also tend to be very portable. They're often made into bite-sized balls, cut into little squares, or shaped with specialized silicone molds, so you can easily take them on the go and have them with you at all times should a fat or hunger emergency strike.

On the other hand, a general keto snack is one that still contains a high amount of fat, as all keto-approved meals and snacks do, but has some more leniency when it comes to protein and carbohydrates. Keto snacks may contain some vegetables or meat, whereas fat bombs typically only contain oils, nuts and nut butters, keto-approved sweeteners, and natural flavors.

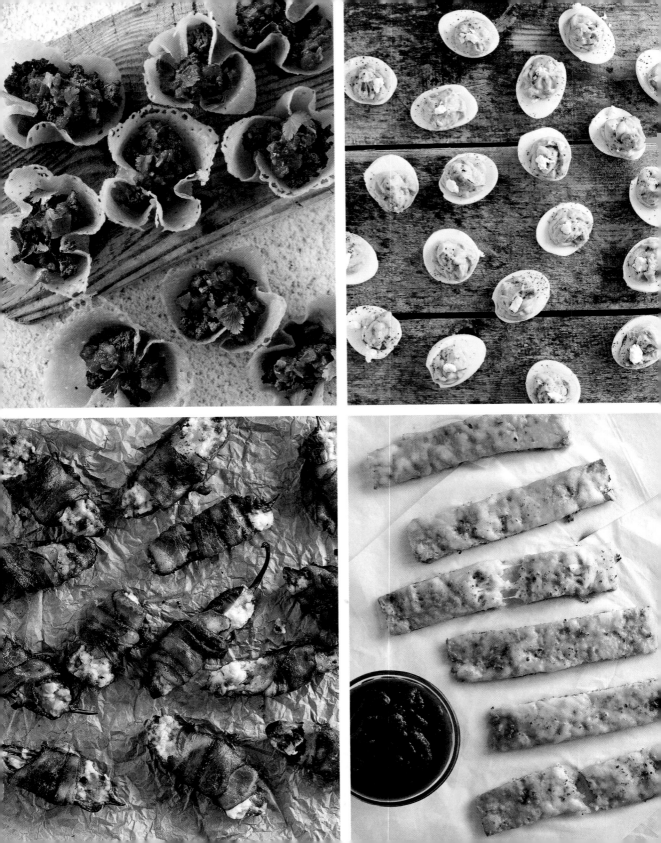

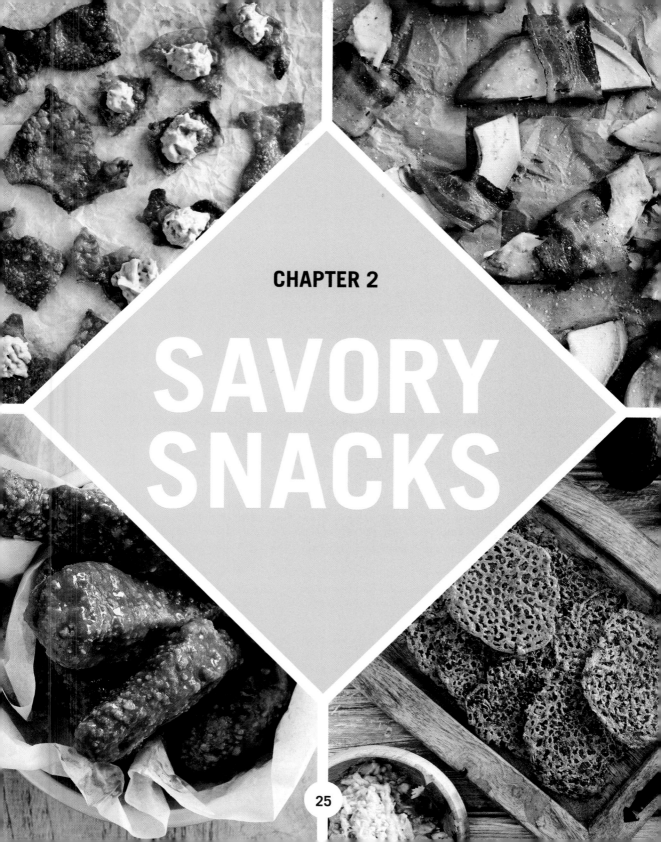

# CHAPTER 2

# SAVORY SNACKS

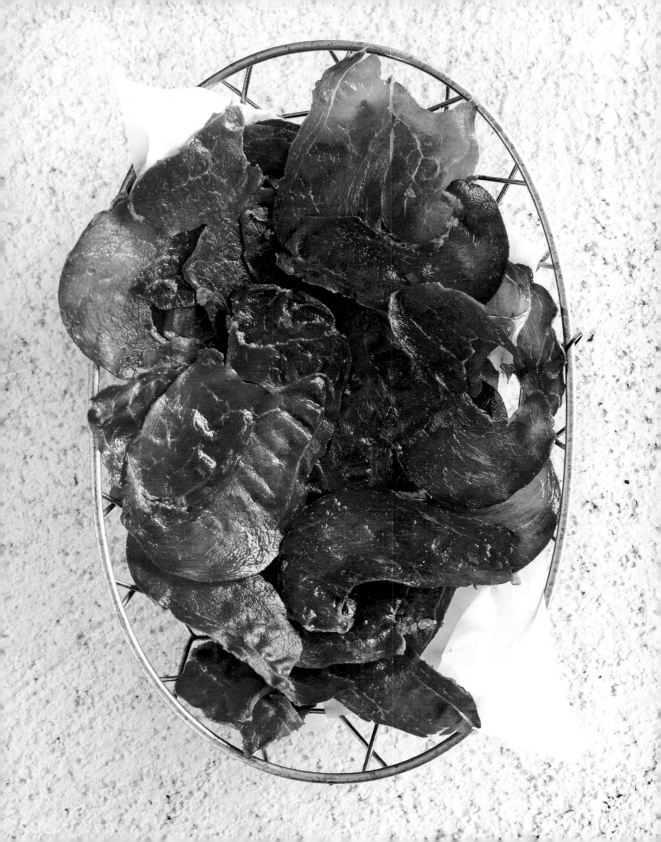

# PROSCIUTTO CHIPS

*These Prosciutto Chips are so simple and delicious; you'll wonder why you never thought of them before. All you need is some prosciutto and an oven.*

**Serves 4**

**12 (1-ounce) slices prosciutto**

**1** Preheat oven to 350°F.

**2** Line a baking sheet with parchment paper and lay prosciutto slices out in a single layer. Bake 12 minutes or until prosciutto is crispy.

**3** Let cool completely before eating.

**Per Serving**
Calories: 250 | Fat: 19.0 g | Protein: 18.0 g | Sodium: 340 mg | Fiber: 0.0 g | Carbohydrates: 2.0 g | Net Carbohydrates: 2.0 g | Sugar: 0.0 g

### A Little about Prosciutto

Prosciutto is made from the hind leg of a pig, or the ham. It is sliced thinly and rubbed with salt, which draws out the moisture to concentrate the flavor. This process, called curing, can take from a few months to several years.

# DEVILED EGGS

*Deviled eggs are a staple at any party, and they make the perfect ketogenic diet snack. Whip some up and store them in your refrigerator for when you need some fat and protein in a hurry.*

**Serves 6**

6 large hard-boiled eggs
¼ cup keto-approved mayonnaise
1 teaspoon white vinegar
1 teaspoon dry mustard
½ teaspoon salt
¼ teaspoon black pepper
⅛ teaspoon smoked paprika

**1** Peel eggs and cut in half lengthwise. Scoop out egg yolks and put in a small mixing bowl.

**2** Mash yolks with a fork, then add mayonnaise, vinegar, mustard, salt, and pepper. Continue to mash until combined.

**3** Divide mixture into 12 equal portions and fill each egg white half. Sprinkle with paprika.

**Per Serving**
Calories: 146 | Fat: 12.5 g | Protein: 6.4 g | Sodium: 305 mg | Fiber: 0.1 g | Carbohydrates: 0.8 g | Net Carbohydrates: 0.7 g | Sugar: 0.6 g

# BUFFALO CAULIFLOWER BITES

*These Buffalo Cauliflower Bites give you all the flavor of traditional buffalo wings with minimal carbohydrates. They'll be a hit even with those not following a ketogenic diet. Serve these bites with a ranch dipping sauce.*

**Serves 6**

1 cup almond meal

1 teaspoon granulated garlic

½ teaspoon dried parsley

½ teaspoon salt

1 large egg

1 large head cauliflower, cut into bite-sized florets

½ cup Frank's RedHot sauce

¼ cup ghee

**1** Preheat oven to 400°F. Line a baking sheet with parchment paper.

**2** Combine almond meal, garlic, parsley, and salt in a large sealable plastic bag and shake to mix.

**3** Whisk egg in a large bowl. Add cauliflower and toss to coat completely.

**4** Transfer cauliflower to bag filled with almond meal mixture and toss to coat.

**5** Arrange cauliflower in a single layer on baking sheet and bake 30 minutes or until softened and slightly browned.

**6** While cauliflower is baking, combine hot sauce and ghee in a small saucepan over low heat.

**7** When cauliflower is cooked, combine cauliflower with hot sauce mixture in a large mixing bowl and toss to coat.

**Per Serving**
Calories: 209 | Fat: 19.5 g | Protein: 5.9 g | Sodium: 830 mg | Fiber: 2.8 g | Carbohydrates: 6.4 g | Net Carbohydrates: 3.6 g | Sugar: 1.5 g

# CHEESY CAULIFLOWER BREADSTICKS

*You can easily transform these into pizza cauliflower breadsticks by adding some no-sugar-added pizza sauce to the cauliflower before adding cheese and then following the rest of the recipe as written.*

**Serves 6**

1½ cups riced cauliflower
½ teaspoon dried oregano
½ teaspoon dried thyme
¼ teaspoon ground sage
¼ teaspoon black pepper
¾ cup shredded mozzarella cheese
¾ cup shredded Cheddar cheese
2 large eggs, lightly beaten

**1** Preheat oven to 450°F. Lightly grease a rimmed baking sheet.

**2** Place cauliflower in a small microwave-safe bowl and microwave on high 5–6 minutes or until softened. Allow cauliflower to cool and then transfer to a nut milk bag or cheesecloth and squeeze out excess moisture.

**3** Transfer drained cauliflower to a medium mixing bowl.

**4** Add oregano, thyme, sage, and pepper and mix to thoroughly combine.

**5** Combine cheeses in a small bowl. Then add ⅓ cup combined cheese and the eggs to the cauliflower mixture and mix to combine. Drain any excess liquid.

**6** Transfer cauliflower to baking sheet and press into a rectangle, about ⅓" thick.

**7** Bake 15 minutes, remove from heat, sprinkle remaining cheese on top, and bake 5 more minutes or until cheese is melted and bubbly.

**8** Cool 5 minutes and slice into strips.

**Per Serving**
Calories: 75 | Fat: 4.3 g | Protein: 5.7 g | Sodium: 116 mg | Fiber: 0.6 g | Carbohydrates: 1.6 g | Net Carbohydrates: 1.0 g | Sugar: 0.7 g

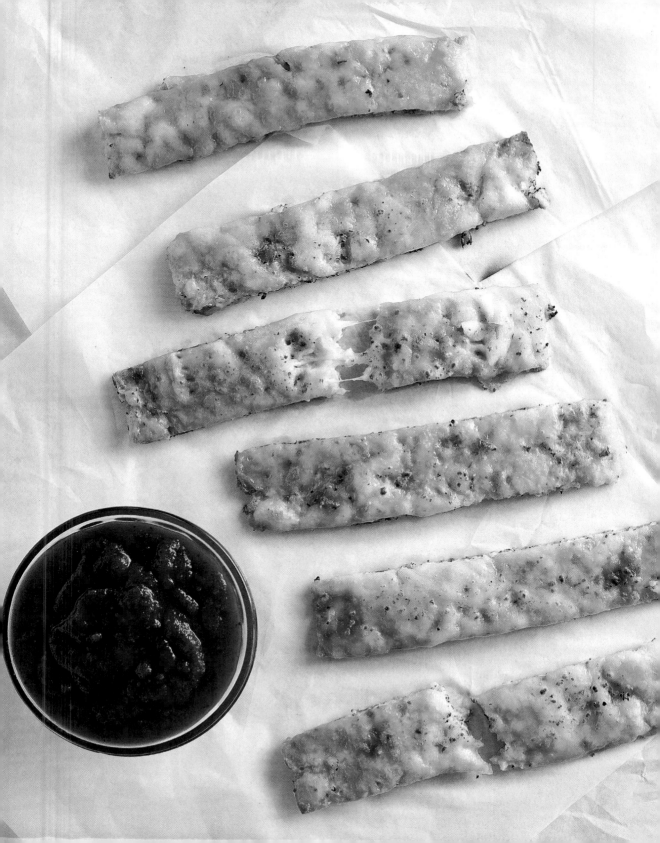

# CAULIFLOWER LATKES

*Traditional latkes are made with shredded potato, which doesn't have a place in the ketogenic diet. This version can satisfy a latke craving while keeping you within your carbohydrate goals for the day.*

**Serves 6**

4 cups cauliflower florets
1 tablespoon olive oil
¾ cup minced yellow onion
½ cup almond meal
2 large eggs, lightly beaten
2 tablespoons chopped fresh parsley
1 teaspoon salt
½ teaspoon black pepper
2 tablespoons coconut oil

**1** Place cauliflower florets in the bowl of a food processor and pulse until "rice" is formed.

**2** Transfer to a medium microwave-safe bowl and microwave on high 2 minutes. Allow to cool and then transfer cauliflower to a nut milk bag or cheesecloth and squeeze out excess moisture. Put drained cauliflower back in bowl.

**3** Add olive oil to a medium skillet and heat over medium heat. Add onions and cook until caramelized, about 5 minutes. Transfer onions to bowl with cauliflower.

**4** Add remaining ingredients except coconut oil to bowl and use your hands to mix thoroughly. Form mixture into patties and set aside.

**5** Heat coconut oil in the same skillet over medium-high heat. Add latke patties and cook until golden brown, about 3 minutes on each side.

**6** Serve with topping of your choice.

## What's a Latke?

Latkes are potato pancakes that are traditionally served during Hanukkah—or the Festival of Lights. They're usually served with sour cream or applesauce, but for a ketogenic diet, you'll want to stick with sour cream if you need something to dip them in.

**Per Serving**
Calories: 162 | Fat: 12.7 g | Protein: 5.7 g | Sodium: 433 mg | Fiber: 2.9 g | Carbohydrates: 7.7 g | Net Carbohydrates: 4.8 g | Sugar: 2.6 g

# CAULIFLOWER CUPS

*These Cauliflower Cups are designed to be a snack, but you can turn them into breakfast by adding more eggs to the mixture and cooking them in a regular muffin pan.*

**Serves 6**

1½ cups cauliflower rice
¼ cup diced onion
½ cup shredded pepper jack cheese
½ teaspoon dried oregano
½ teaspoon dried basil
½ teaspoon salt
1 large egg, lightly beaten

**1** Preheat oven to 350°F.

**2** Combine all ingredients in a large mixing bowl and stir to incorporate.

**3** Scoop mixture into the wells of a mini muffin tin and pack lightly.

**4** Bake 30 minutes or until cups start to crisp. Allow to cool slightly and remove from tin.

**Per Serving**
Calories: 60 | Fat: 3.9 g | Protein: 4.3 g | Sodium: 276 mg | Fiber: 0.7 g | Carbohydrates: 1.8 g | Net Carbohydrates: 1.1 g | Sugar: 0.9 g

## Ricing Your Cauliflower

Cauliflower "rice" has become such a staple in the ketogenic and low-carb communities that companies are starting to catch on and offer cauliflower already riced for you. You can find it in the freezer or refrigerated section of your grocery store. If you can't find pre-riced cauliflower, you can make your own by putting cauliflower florets in a food processor and pulsing until a "rice" forms. Be careful not to over-pulse, though, or you'll end up with mashed cauliflower.

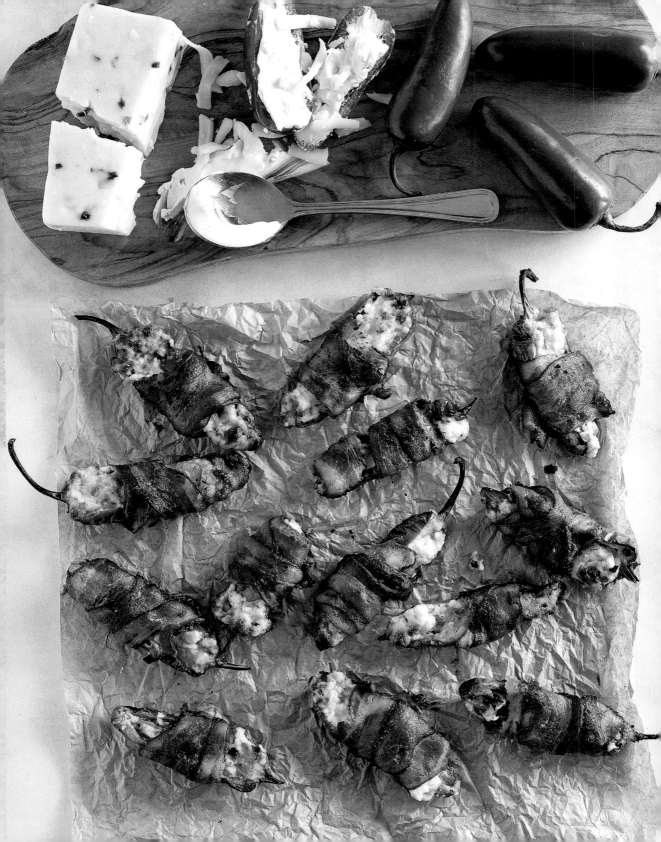

# JALAPEÑO POPPERS

*To double the yield of this recipe, cut the jalapeños in half and wrap each half in a half piece of bacon.*

**Serves 4**

8 medium jalapeño peppers
4 ounces (½ cup) cream cheese, softened
½ cup shredded pepper jack cheese
8 slices no-sugar-added bacon

**1** Preheat oven to 425°F. Line a cookie sheet with aluminum foil.

**2** Cut about ⅓ of each pepper off lengthwise to make a little pocket for filling. Scoop out seeds.

**3** Mix cream cheese and pepper jack cheese together in a small bowl. Divide filling into 8 equal portions and stuff each pepper with cheese filling.

**4** Wrap each pepper in bacon. Lay flat on cookie sheet and bake 15–20 minutes or until bacon is crispy.

**Per Serving**
Calories: 255 | Fat: 19.3 g | Protein: 11.8 g | Sodium: 558 mg | Fiber: 0.8 g | Carbohydrates: 3.3 g | Net Carbohydrates: 2.5 g | Sugar: 2.2 g

## Turn Up the Heat

The capsaicin in chili peppers is thermogenic, which means it generates heat by increasing the metabolism of adipose (fat) tissue. Eating capsaicin-rich foods may help stimulate the body's ability to burn fat.

# STUFFED OLIVES

*You can use any type of olives you want for this recipe, but green olives have a tangy flavor that complements the blue cheese wonderfully.*

**Serves 8**

¼ cup blue cheese crumbles
2 ounces (¼ cup) cream cheese, softened
24 large green olives

**1** Beat blue cheese and cream cheese together in a small bowl until light and fluffy.

**2** Fill each olive with 1 teaspoon filling. Serve at room temperature.

**Per Serving**
Calories: 54 | Fat: 4.6 g | Protein: 1.4 g | Sodium: 171 mg | Fiber: 0.4 g | Carbohydrates: 1.2 g | Net Carbohydrates: 0.8 g | Sugar: 0.3 g

# PIZZA DIP

*You can tailor this Pizza Dip to your liking by adding other keto-friendly ingredients like pepperoni, olives, or green peppers. Serve this dip with zucchini slices or Keto Crackers (see recipe in this chapter).*

**Serves 6**

1 (8-ounce) package cream cheese, softened
½ cup plain Greek yogurt
1 teaspoon dried oregano
¼ teaspoon dried basil
½ teaspoon granulated onion
½ teaspoon granulated garlic
¾ cup no-sugar-added pizza sauce
½ cup shredded mozzarella cheese
¼ teaspoon salt
¼ teaspoon black pepper

**1** Preheat oven to 350°F.

**2** Combine cream cheese, yogurt, oregano, basil, onion, and garlic in a medium bowl and mix with a handheld mixer until combined. Spread mixture into the bottom of an 8" × 8" baking pan.

**3** Spread pizza sauce on top of cream cheese mixture, sprinkle with mozzarella cheese, and top with salt and pepper.

**4** Bake covered 15 minutes. Remove cover and bake an additional 10 minutes or until cheese is golden and bubbly.

### Homemade Pizza Sauce

If you can't find pizza sauce without added sugar or you want to quickly whip up your own, you can combine 1 (8-ounce) can tomato sauce with 1 teaspoon minced garlic, 1 teaspoon dried oregano, and ½ teaspoon dried basil in a medium bowl and use that.

**Per Serving**
Calories: 200 | Fat: 14.9 g | Protein: 6.6 g | Sodium: 424 mg | Fiber: 0.7 g | Carbohydrates: 6.0 g | Net Carbohydrates: 5.3 g | Sugar: 3.1 g

# GUACAMOLE

*Guacamole is a ketogenic diet staple. Eat it with some celery stalks, put it on top of your taco bowls, or spoon it right out of the bowl.*

**Serves 4**

3 large avocados
Juice from 1 medium lime
2 large Roma tomatoes, diced
2 cloves garlic, minced
¼ cup chopped fresh cilantro
¼ cup chopped red onion
½ teaspoon salt
½ teaspoon black pepper

**1** Cut avocados in half lengthwise, remove the pits, and scoop them out of the skin and into a medium bowl. Add lime juice. Use a fork to mash avocado and lime together, leaving some chunks intact.

**2** Add tomatoes, garlic, cilantro, onion, salt, and pepper. Mash with a fork until combined.

**Per Serving**
Calories: 186 | Fat: 14.1 g | Protein: 2.7 g | Sodium: 301 mg | Fiber: 7.8 g | Carbohydrates: 12.9 g | Net Carbohydrates: 5.1 g | Sugar: 2.1 g

## Amazing Avocado

About 77 percent of the calories in an avocado come from fat, which makes it one of the fattiest foods in the world. Ounce for ounce avocados also contain more potassium than bananas, so they're especially beneficial during the initial stages of a ketogenic diet when you're losing water weight and electrolytes.

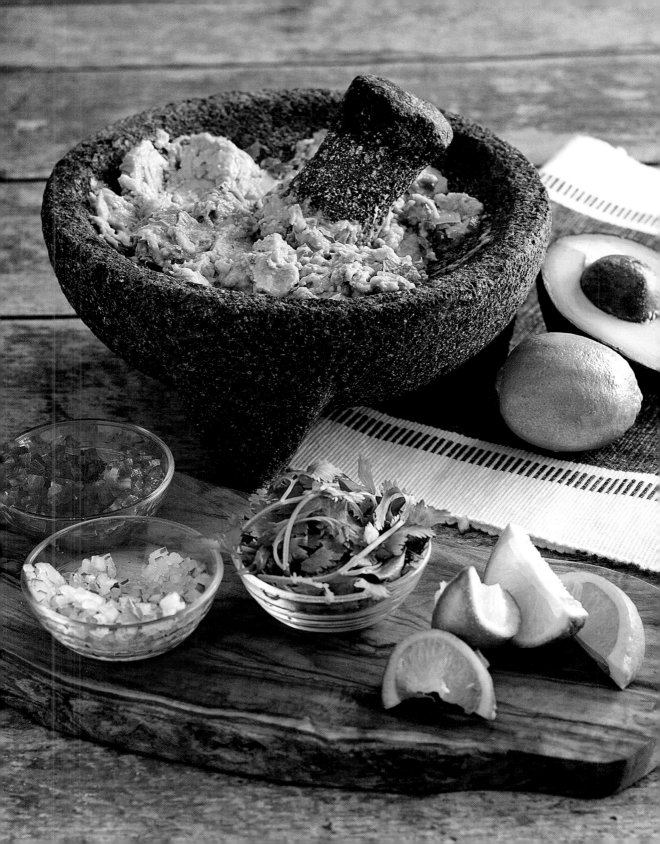

# MEATLOAF MUFFINS

*These Meatloaf Muffins are the perfect on-the-go keto snack. You can switch it up by making them with ground chicken, ground turkey, ground pork, or a combination of any of those. Serve these with no-sugar-added ketchup.*

**Serves 6**

1 pound ground beef
1 cup chopped spinach
1 large egg, lightly beaten
½ cup shredded mozzarella cheese
¼ cup grated Parmesan cheese
¼ cup chopped yellow onion
2 tablespoons seeded and minced jalapeño pepper

**1** Preheat oven to 350°F. Lightly grease each well of a muffin tin.

**2** Combine all ingredients in large bowl and use your hands to mix.

**3** Scoop an equal portion of meat mixture into each muffin tin and press down lightly. Bake 45 minutes or until internal temperature reaches 165°F.

**Per Serving**
Calories: 198 | Fat: 13.8 g | Protein: 11.9 g | Sodium: 180 mg | Fiber: 0.3 g | Carbohydrates: 1.8 g | Net Carbohydrates: 1.5 g | Sugar: 0.5 g

# MACADAMIA NUT HUMMUS

*This recipe requires you to soak the macadamia nuts before using them. If you don't soak the nuts, the texture won't be right, so plan for this extra time when making this hummus. Serve with cucumber or zucchini slices.*

**Serves 6**

1 cup macadamia nuts, soaked
3 cloves garlic
3 tablespoons lemon juice
2 tablespoons water
3 tablespoons tahini
½ teaspoon salt
¼ teaspoon black pepper

Combine all ingredients in a food processor and process until smooth.

**Per Serving**
Calories: 208 | Fat: 20.0 g | Protein: 3.2 g | Sodium: 203 mg | Fiber: 2.7 g | Carbohydrates: 5.8 g | Net Carbohydrates: 3.1 g | Sugar: 1.3 g

## How to Soak Macadamia Nuts

To soak macadamia nuts, try this: Put 1 cup macadamia nuts in a small glass bowl and cover with 2 cups filtered water and a pinch of sea salt. Cover with a thin towel and keep the soaking nuts at room temperature for 2 hours. (Other types of nuts, like almonds, require a longer soaking time.)

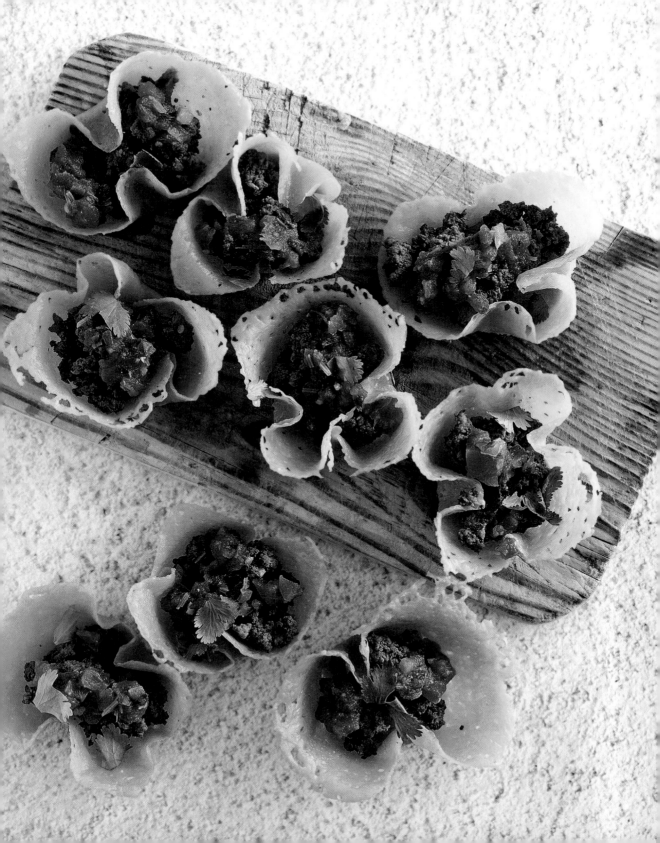

# TACO CUPS

*You can make these Taco Cups your own by adding any keto-friendly toppings you want. Olives, avocados, and chopped red onions are excellent additions.*

**Serves 4**

1 tablespoon chili powder

1½ teaspoons ground cumin

½ teaspoon ground paprika

1 teaspoon salt

1 teaspoon black pepper

¼ teaspoon dried oregano

¼ teaspoon crushed red pepper flakes

¼ teaspoon granulated garlic

¼ teaspoon granulated onion

1 pound 75% lean ground beef

8 (1-ounce) slices sharp Cheddar cheese

½ cup no-sugar-added salsa

¼ cup chopped cilantro

3 tablespoons Frank's RedHot sauce

**1** Preheat oven to 375°F. Line a baking sheet with parchment paper.

**2** Combine spices in a small bowl and stir to mix. Cook ground beef in a medium skillet over medium-high heat. When beef is almost done cooking, add spice mixture and stir to coat completely. Remove from heat and set aside.

**3** Arrange Cheddar cheese slices on lined baking sheet. Bake in preheated oven 5 minutes or until starting to brown. Allow to cool 3 minutes and then peel from baking sheet and transfer each slice to the well of a muffin tin, forming a cup. Allow to cool.

**4** Scoop equal amounts of meat into each cup and top with 1 tablespoon of salsa. Sprinkle cilantro and hot sauce on top.

**Per Serving**
Calories: 457 | Fat: 32.2 g | Protein: 25.7 g | Sodium: 1,519 mg | Fiber: 1.5 g | Carbohydrates: 5.0 g | Net Carbohydrates: 3.5 g | Sugar: 0.4 g

# KETO CRACKERS

*With this recipe, you don't have to miss crackers on a ketogenic diet. They're the perfect pairing for any of the keto-friendly hummuses or dips.*

**Serves 6**

1 cup grated Parmesan cheese
1 cup shredded Cheddar cheese
2 ounces (¼ cup) cream cheese, softened
1 cup almond flour
1 large egg, lightly beaten
¾ teaspoon salt
1 teaspoon granulated garlic
½ teaspoon dried rosemary

**1** Preheat oven to 450°F. Line a baking sheet with parchment paper.

**2** Combine Parmesan cheese, Cheddar cheese, cream cheese, and almond flour in a medium saucepan and heat over low heat. Stir constantly until cheeses have just melted. Remove from heat and allow to cool.

**3** Once cheese mixture has adequately cooled, add egg and spices and stir to combine. Mixture should be doughlike.

**4** Place dough between two sheets of parchment paper and roll out into a rectangle. Cut the dough into crackers, approximately 1½" squares, and arrange in a single layer on the baking sheet.

**5** Bake 12 minutes, turning crackers over once during cooking. If after 12 minutes crackers are not crispy, continue baking until they reach your desired level of doneness.

**6** Allow to cool slightly before eating.

## Make Them Your Own

You can make these Keto Crackers with any combination of flavors by using any of your favorite herbs and spices in place of the garlic and rosemary. Try sage and thyme or granulated garlic and granulated onion.

**Per Serving**
Calories: 298 | Fat: 22.3 g | Protein: 15.0 g | Sodium: 758 mg | Fiber: 2.1 g | Carbohydrates: 7.5 g | Net Carbohydrates: 5.4 g | Sugar: 1.1 g

# KETO ENERGY BALLS

*Typically, energy balls are made from oats and dried fruits, which don't have a place on a ketogenic diet. These energy balls are just as quick, easy, and delicious, but with significantly fewer carbohydrates.*

**Serves 6**

2 tablespoons grass-fed butter

⅔ cup no-sugar-added creamy cashew butter

1 cup unsweetened shredded coconut

5 drops liquid stevia

¼ cup crushed cashews

**1** Heat butter in a small saucepan over low heat. Once melted, add cashew butter and stir until smooth.

**2** Stir in remaining ingredients.

**3** Line a baking sheet with parchment paper and drop mixture by rounded spoonfuls in a single layer.

**4** Freeze 1 hour. Remove from freezer and transfer to an airtight container. Store in the refrigerator until ready to eat.

**Per Serving**
Calories: 325 | Fat: 28.0 g | Protein: 6.8 g | Sodium: 16 mg | Fiber: 3.4 g | Carbohydrates: 13.4 g | Net Carbohydrates: 10.0 g | Sugar: 1.2 g

# BACON-WRAPPED AVOCADO BITES

*Bacon and avocado may not sound like a good combination, but don't knock it till you try it: the salty, crispy bacon and smooth, creamy avocado make the perfect pair.*

**Serves 4**

2 large avocados, peeled and pitted
8 slices no-sugar-added bacon
½ teaspoon garlic salt

**1** Preheat oven to 425°F. Line a cookie sheet with parchment paper.

**2** Cut each avocado into 8 equal-sized slices, making 16 slices total.

**3** Cut each piece of bacon in half. Wrap a half slice of bacon around each piece of avocado. Sprinkle with garlic salt.

**4** Place avocado on cookie sheet and bake 15 minutes. Turn oven to broil and continue to cook another 2–3 minutes until bacon becomes crispy.

### Precook Your Bacon

If you cook avocado too long, it can turn bitter. To avoid this, you can shorten the cooking time of this recipe by slightly precooking the bacon—enough that it's partially cooked but still bendable—and then wrapping it around the avocado and putting it in the oven.

**Per Serving**
Calories: 202 | Fat: 15.5 g | Protein: 7.1 g | Sodium: 605 mg | Fiber: 4.6 g | Carbohydrates: 6.1 g | Net Carbohydrates: 1.5 g | Sugar: 0.2 g

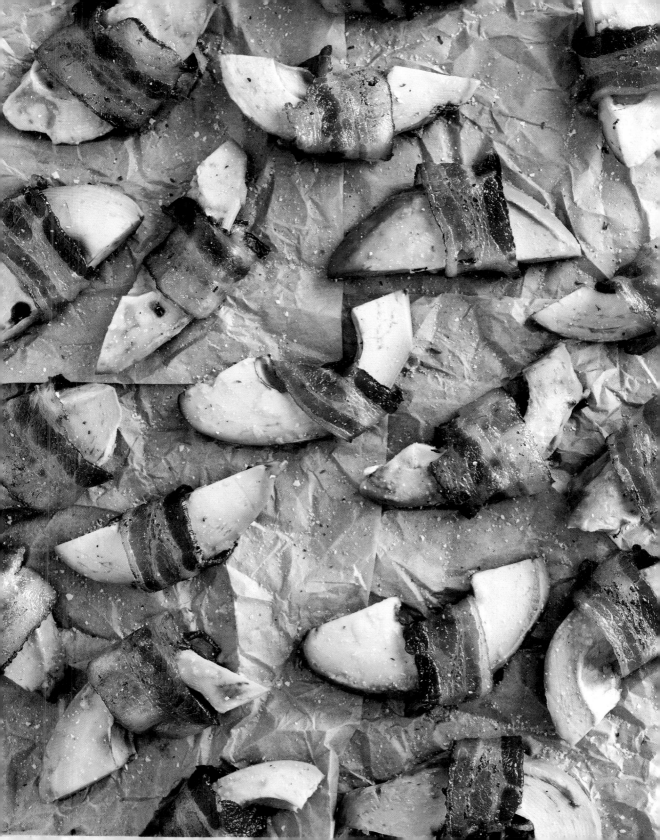

# BUFFALO CHICKEN DIP

*This Buffalo Chicken Dip goes exceptionally well with celery sticks. You can also serve it with raw sliced zucchini, another versatile vegetable with minimal flavor and a big crunch.*

**Serves 6**

**1 (8-ounce) package cream cheese**
**½ cup Frank's RedHot sauce**
**¼ cup full-fat canned coconut milk**
**1½ cups shredded cooked chicken**
**¾ cup shredded mozzarella cheese, divided**
**½ cup blue cheese crumbles**

**1** Add cream cheese to a medium saucepan and heat over medium-low heat until melted. Stir in hot sauce and coconut milk.

**2** When combined, add chicken until heated through.

**3** Remove from heat and stir in ½ cup mozzarella cheese and blue cheese crumbles.

**4** Transfer to an 8" × 8" baking dish and sprinkle remaining mozzarella cheese on top. Bake 15 minutes or until cheese is bubbly. Serve warm.

**Per Serving**
Calories: 287 | Fat: 20.9 g | Protein: 16.7 g | Sodium: 995 mg | Fiber: 0.0 g | Carbohydrates: 2.4 g | Net Carbohydrates: 2.4 g | Sugar: 1.4 g

**Make It Ranch**

If you don't like blue cheese, you can omit the blue cheese crumbles and use ½ cup of Ranch Dip (see recipe in this chapter) in its place or just omit it completely.

# AVOCADO HUMMUS

*Like the Macadamia Nut Hummus (see recipe in this chapter), this Avocado Hummus requires you to soak the macadamia nuts before putting this recipe together. Keep that in mind when working this into your meal plan. Serve this hummus with cucumber slices or Keto Crackers (see recipe in this chapter).*

**Serves 6**

1¼ cups macadamia nuts, soaked
1 large avocado, peeled and pitted
3 cloves garlic
2 tablespoons lime juice
2 tablespoons tahini
1 tablespoon olive oil
1 teaspoon salt
½ teaspoon black pepper
3–4 tablespoons water

**1** Combine all ingredients, except water, in a food processor and process until combined.

**2** Add water 1 tablespoon at a time until you reach desired consistency.

**Per Serving**
Calories: 291 | Fat: 28.1 g | Protein: 3.6 g | Sodium: 396 mg | Fiber: 4.5 g | Carbohydrates: 7.9 g | Net Carbohydrates: 3.4 g | Sugar: 1.5 g

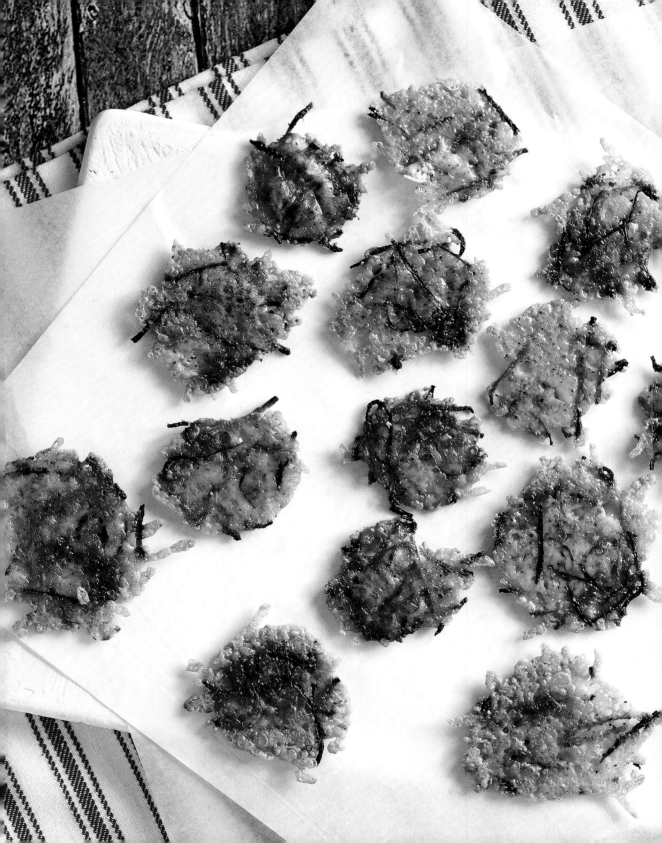

# PARMESAN VEGETABLE CRISPS

*This simple twist on the Parmesan crisp introduces added texture and a mild sweetness while offering additional fiber too. Of course, the added colors of the vegetables make this crisp a beauty for the eyes to feast on before you taste it. Enjoy these as is or with fat-bomb dips and spreads.*

**Serves 4**

¾ cup shredded zucchini
¼ cup shredded carrots
2 cups freshly shredded Parmesan cheese
1 tablespoon olive oil
¼ teaspoon black pepper

**1** Preheat oven to 375°F. Prepare a cookie sheet with parchment paper or a Silpat mat.

**2** Wrap shredded vegetables in a paper towel and wring out excess moisture.

**3** Mix all ingredients in a medium bowl until thoroughly combined.

**4** Place tablespoon-sized mounds onto prepared cookie sheet.

**5** Bake 7–10 minutes until lightly browned.

**6** Let cool 2–3 minutes and remove from cookie sheet.

## Zucchini: A Kitchen Staple

It's no secret that the right vegetables are an important part of any healthy diet. Zucchini is a fantastic choice for high-fat, low-carbohydrate diets because it has a low carbohydrate content (low glycemic index) and it's full of potassium, a crucial mineral for heart health. Besides that, it also makes a fantastic substitute for pasta lovers looking for low-carbohydrate alternatives.

**Per Serving**
Calories: 206 | Fat: 14.1 g | Protein: 15.8 g | Sodium: 686 mg | Fiber: 0.7 g | Carbohydrates: 3.6 g | Net Carbohydrates: 2.9 g | Sugar: 1.9 g

# SPICY SHRIMP AND CHEESE DIP

*Cooking tip: if the dip is too thick, add coconut milk or heavy cream in half-cup increments until it's the consistency you like. This dip is heavenly with the addition of 1 cup chopped cooked scallops.*

**Serves 12**

2 slices no-sugar-added bacon

2 medium yellow onions, peeled and diced

2 cloves garlic, minced

1 cup popcorn shrimp (not the breaded kind), cooked

1 medium tomato, diced

3 cups shredded Monterey jack cheese

¼ teaspoon Frank's RedHot sauce

¼ teaspoon cayenne pepper

¼ teaspoon black pepper

**1** Cook the bacon in a medium skillet over medium heat until crisp, about 5–10 minutes. Keep grease in pan. Lay the bacon on a paper towel to cool. When cool, crumble the bacon with your fingers.

**2** Add the onion and garlic to the bacon drippings in the skillet and sauté over medium-low heat until they are soft and fragrant, about 10 minutes.

**3** Combine all the ingredients in a slow cooker; stir well. Cook covered on low setting 1–2 hours or until cheese is fully melted.

**Per Serving**
Calories: 156 | Fat: 9.2 g | Protein: 14.1 g | Sodium: 463 mg | Fiber: 0.5 g | Carbohydrates: 3.0 g | Net Carbohydrates: 2.5 g | Sugar: 1.2 g

# GARLIC AND BACON DIP

*This dip is excellent with keto-friendly veggies like celery or sliced cucumbers, or you can combine it with Keto Crackers (see recipe in this chapter).*

**Serves 6**

8 slices no-sugar-added bacon
2 cups chopped spinach
1 (8-ounce) package cream cheese, softened
¼ cup full-fat sour cream
¼ cup plain full-fat Greek yogurt
2 tablespoons chopped fresh parsley
1 tablespoon lemon juice
6 cloves roasted garlic, mashed
1 teaspoon salt
½ teaspoon black pepper
½ cup grated Parmesan cheese

**1** Preheat oven to 350°F.

**2** Cook bacon in a medium skillet over medium heat until crispy. Remove bacon from pan and set aside on a plate lined with paper towels.

**3** Add spinach to hot pan and cook until wilted. Remove from heat and set aside.

**4** To a medium bowl, add cream cheese, sour cream, yogurt, parsley, lemon juice, garlic, salt, and pepper and beat with a handheld mixer until combined.

**5** Roughly chop bacon and stir into cream cheese mixture. Stir in spinach and Parmesan cheese.

**6** Transfer to an 8" × 8" baking pan and bake 30 minutes or until hot and bubbly.

## Roasted Garlic Recipe

Roasting garlic brings out a deep flavor that you don't get with raw. Preheat your oven to 400°F. Remove the excess skin from 6 bulbs of garlic and cut ½" off the tips. Line a pie plate with aluminum foil and arrange bulbs in a single layer. Drizzle olive oil on top and wrap bulbs with foil. Roast 30 minutes. Allow to cool and remove cloves from bulb. Store in the refrigerator up to 2 weeks.

**Per Serving**
Calories: 271 | Fat: 20.4 g | Protein: 11.4 g | Sodium: 950 mg | Fiber: 0.4 g | Carbohydrates: 5.3 g | Net Carbohydrates: 4.9 g | Sugar: 2.0 g

# CHEDDAR MEXI-MELT CRISPS

*Another versatile cheese for the low-carbohydrate kitchen is Cheddar, the harder the better. Generally, the harder Cheddars tend to be the sharpest, so if tart and tangy seems like too much, a mild Cheddar will also work for these crisps. Enjoy these crisps as is or with guacamole.*

**Serves 2**

1 cup shredded sharp Cheddar cheese
⅛ teaspoon granulated garlic
⅛ teaspoon chili powder
⅛ teaspoon ground cumin
1/16 teaspoon cayenne pepper
1 tablespoon finely chopped cilantro
1 teaspoon olive oil

**1** Preheat oven to 350°F. Prepare a cookie sheet with parchment paper or a Silpat mat.

**2** Mix all ingredients in a medium bowl until well combined.

**3** Drop by tablespoon-sized portions onto prepared cookie sheet.

**4** Cook 5–7 minutes until edges begin to brown.

**5** Allow to cool 2–3 minutes before removing from cookie sheet with a spatula.

**Per Serving**
Calories: 249 | Fat: 18.8 g | Protein: 13.7 g | Sodium: 368 mg | Fiber: 0.1 g | Carbohydrates: 1.1 g | Net Carbohydrates: 1.0 g | Sugar: 0.2 g

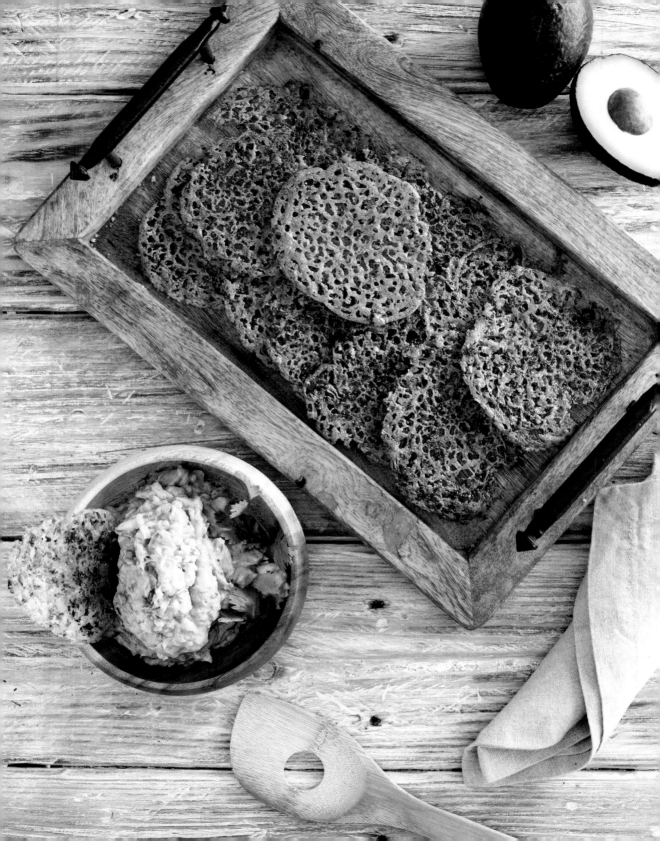

# CHICKEN SKIN CRISPS SATAY

*If you like Thai food, this fat-bomb recipe will absolutely delight you!*

**Makes 6 fat bombs**

**Skin from 3 large chicken thighs**
**2 tablespoons no-sugar-added chunky peanut butter**
**1 tablespoon unsweetened coconut cream**
**1 teaspoon coconut oil**
**1 teaspoon seeded and minced jalapeño pepper**
**¼ clove garlic, minced**
**1 teaspoon coconut aminos**

**1** Preheat oven to 350°F. On a cookie sheet lined with parchment paper, lay out skins as flat as possible.

**2** Bake 12–15 minutes until skins turn light brown and crispy, being careful not to burn them.

**3** Remove skins from cookie sheet and place on a paper towel to cool.

**4** In a small food processor, add peanut butter, coconut cream, coconut oil, jalapeño, garlic, and coconut aminos. Mix until well blended, about 30 seconds.

**5** Cut each crispy chicken skin in 2 pieces.

**6** Place 1 tablespoon peanut sauce on each chicken crisp and serve immediately. If sauce is too runny, refrigerate 2 hours before using.

## Precious Liquid Fat

When you cook the chicken skins, you will end up with a pan full of chicken fat. You can drain that into a glass jar and save it for later. This fat can be stored in the refrigerator for a couple of months, and it can be used in any recipe as a 100 percent dairy-free substitute for butter.

**Per Serving**
Calories: 112 | Fat: 9.9 g | Protein: 3.8 g | Sodium: 30 mg | Fiber: 0.6 g | Carbohydrates: 1.6 g | Net Carbohydrates: 1.0 g | Sugar: 0.2 g

# CRAB RANGOON DIP

*Here is one of the best ways to enjoy a Chinese takeout favorite without the added carbohydrates. This dip is best enjoyed on celery sticks or Parmesan crisps.*

**Serves 4**

1 (8-ounce) package cream cheese, softened to room temperature
2 tablespoons olive oil mayonnaise
1 tablespoon freshly squeezed lemon juice
½ teaspoon sea salt
¼ teaspoon black pepper
2 cloves garlic, minced
2 medium green onions, diced
½ cup shredded Parmesan cheese
4 ounces (about ½ cup) canned white crabmeat

**1** Preheat oven to 350°F.

**2** In a medium bowl, mix cream cheese, mayonnaise, lemon juice, salt, and pepper with a hand blender until well incorporated.

**3** Add garlic, onions, Parmesan cheese, and crabmeat and fold into mixture with a spatula.

**4** Transfer mixture to an oven-safe crock and spread out evenly.

**5** Bake 30–35 minutes until top of dip is slightly browned. Serve warm.

**Per Serving**
Calories: 280 | Fat: 21.0 g | Protein: 12.4 g | Sodium: 778 mg | Fiber: 0.1 g | Carbohydrates: 4.7 g | Net Carbohydrates: 4.6 g | Sugar: 2.3 g

## Allicin and *Allium*

Like shallots, garlic belongs to the genus *Allium*, which also includes onions and leeks. The major compound in garlic, which is called allicin, is responsible for its smell as well as its health benefits, which include boosting the immune system, reducing blood pressure, and reducing the risk of Alzheimer's disease and dementia.

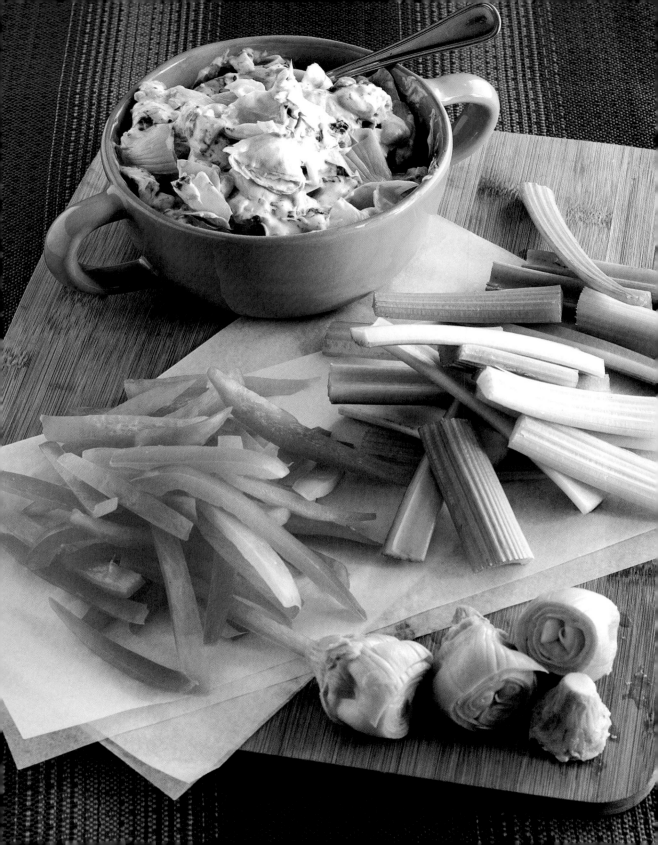

# ARTICHOKE DIP

*For a truly unique appetizer, dollop this dip on top of Parmesan Vegetable Crisps (see recipe in this chapter). Alternatively, use bell pepper strips and celery sticks to scoop and add crunch.*

**Serves 6 as an appetizer**

⅓ cup keto-approved mayonnaise
½ cup grated Parmesan cheese
⅓ cup full-fat sour cream
1 clove garlic, finely minced
1 (6.5-ounce) jar marinated artichoke hearts, chopped into penny-sized pieces

**1** In a medium bowl, combine the mayonnaise, Parmesan cheese, sour cream, and garlic. Mix in the chopped artichoke hearts.

**2** Place the mixture in a slow cooker, cover, and cook on a low setting 1 hour. Mix periodically while it is cooking to ensure that all ingredients combine and meld together.

**Per Serving**
Calories: 173 | Fat: 16.7 g | Protein: 3.3 g | Sodium: 315 mg | Fiber: 0.9 g | Carbohydrates: 2.9 g | Net Carbohydrates: 2.0 g | Sugar: 0.5 g

# PIZZA BITES

*You won't even miss the crust when you try these Pizza Bites. And the best part? They're ready to go in less than 5 minutes.*

**Serves 6**

**24 slices sugar-free pepperoni**
**½ cup keto-approved marinara sauce**
**½ cup shredded mozzarella cheese**

**1** Turn on oven broiler.

**2** Line a baking sheet with parchment paper and lay out pepperoni slices in a single layer.

**3** Put 1 teaspoon marinara sauce on each pepperoni slice and spread out with a spoon. Add 1 teaspoon mozzarella cheese on top of marinara.

**4** Put baking sheet in the oven and broil 3 minutes or until cheese is melted and slightly brown.

**5** Remove from baking sheet and transfer to a paper towel–lined baking sheet to absorb excess grease.

**Per Serving**
Calories: 82 | Fat: 5.4 g | Protein: 4.2 g | Sodium: 282 mg | Fiber: 0.3 g | Carbohydrates: 2.2 g | Net Carbohydrates: 1.9 g | Sugar: 0.8 g

# BACON-WRAPPED CHICKEN BITES

*Serve these Bacon-Wrapped Chicken Bites with a side of Ranch Dip (see recipe in this chapter) to increase both the flavor and the fat content.*

**Serves 6**

¾ **pound boneless, skinless chicken breast, cut into 1" cubes**

½ **teaspoon salt**

½ **teaspoon black pepper**

**5 slices no-sugar-added bacon**

**1** Preheat oven to 375°F.

**2** Toss chicken with salt and pepper.

**3** Cut each slice of bacon into 3 pieces and wrap each piece of chicken in a piece of bacon. Secure with a toothpick.

**4** Put wrapped chicken on a broiler rack and bake 30 minutes, turning over halfway through cooking. Turn oven to broil and broil 3–4 minutes or until bacon is crispy.

**Per Serving**
Calories: 103 | Fat: 3.9 g | Protein: 16.1 g | Sodium: 361 mg | Fiber: 0.1 g | Carbohydrates: 0.2 g | Net Carbohydrates: 0.1 g | Sugar: 0.0 g

# CHICKEN SKIN CRISPS WITH SPICY AVOCADO CREAM

*Sometimes a bit of spice is a great complement to the creaminess of an ingredient. That makes for a well-balanced recipe.*

**Makes 6 fat bombs**

**Skin from 3 large chicken thighs**
**¼ medium avocado, peeled and pitted**
**3 tablespoons full-fat sour cream**
**½ medium jalapeño pepper, seeded and finely chopped**
**½ teaspoon sea salt**

**1** Preheat oven to 350°F. On a cookie sheet lined with parchment paper lay out skins as flat as possible.

**2** Bake 12–15 minutes until skins turn light brown and crispy, being careful not to burn them.

**3** Remove skins from cookie sheet and place on a paper towel to cool.

**4** In a small bowl, combine avocado, sour cream, jalapeño, and salt.

**5** Mix with a fork until well blended.

**6** Cut each crispy chicken skin in 2 pieces.

**7** Place 1 tablespoon avocado mix on each chicken crisp and serve immediately.

**Per Serving**
Calories: 86 | Fat: 7.5 g | Protein: 2.6 g | Sodium: 145 mg | Fiber: 0.4 g | Carbohydrates: 0.7 g | Net Carbohydrates: 0.3 g | Sugar: 0.2 g

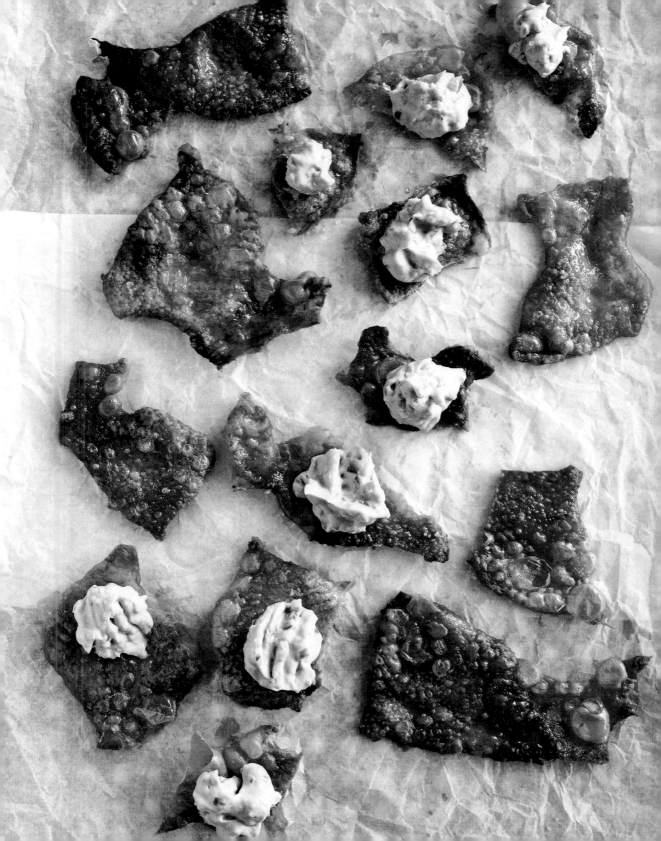

# CHEESY MEATBALLS

*These meatballs freeze well, so feel free to double up the batch when you're making them. You can store them in the freezer after cooking and thaw out a few for a quick, easy-to-eat snack whenever you need it.*

**Serves 6 (makes 24 meatballs)**

1 pound 75% lean ground beef

1 pound 72% lean ground pork

⅓ cup shredded Parmesan cheese

1 teaspoon granulated garlic

1 teaspoon granulated onion

1 teaspoon salt

1 teaspoon black pepper

8 ounces mozzarella cheese, cut into small cubes

1 tablespoon olive oil

**1** Preheat oven to 350°F.

**2** Combine beef, pork, Parmesan cheese, garlic, onion, salt, and pepper in a small bowl. Mix until thoroughly combined.

**3** Divide beef mixture into 24 equal-sized portions and roughly shape into balls. Push a cube of mozzarella cheese into the center of each meatball and reshape to make sure cheese is completely covered.

**4** Heat olive oil in a large skillet over medium heat. Add meatballs to hot oil and brown on all sides (they don't have to be cooked through).

**5** Arrange meatballs on a baking sheet in a single layer and bake 30 minutes, turning over once while cooking.

**6** Remove from oven and serve warm.

**Per Serving**
Calories: 492 | Fat: 34.7 g | Protein: 34.7 g | Sodium: 793 mg | Fiber: 0.2 g | Carbohydrates: 2.6 g | Net Carbohydrates: 2.4 g | Sugar: 0.5 g

# TUNA SALAD AND CUCUMBER BITES

*These bites are an easy snack that's good on the go. Give yourself a little variety by using canned chicken or canned salmon in place of tuna.*

**Serves 4**

2 (5-ounce) cans tuna packed in water, drained

2 large hard-boiled eggs, peeled and chopped

½ cup keto-approved mayonnaise

½ teaspoon salt

½ teaspoon black pepper

2 teaspoons goat cheese

1 medium cucumber, cut into rounds

**1** Put tuna in a medium bowl with chopped eggs, mayonnaise, salt, and pepper. Mash with a fork until combined.

**2** Spread an equal amount of goat cheese on each cucumber slice and top with tuna salad mixture.

**Per Serving**
Calories: 341 | Fat: 29.7 g | Protein: 18.3 g | Sodium: 714 mg | Fiber: 0.3 g | Carbohydrates: 1.1 g | Net Carbohydrates: 0.8 g | Sugar: 0.7 g

## Cool As a Cucumber

Cucumbers are 96 percent water, so they not only provide a good vehicle for getting in your protein and fat, but they also help keep you hydrated. The water in cucumbers helps flush out toxins as well.

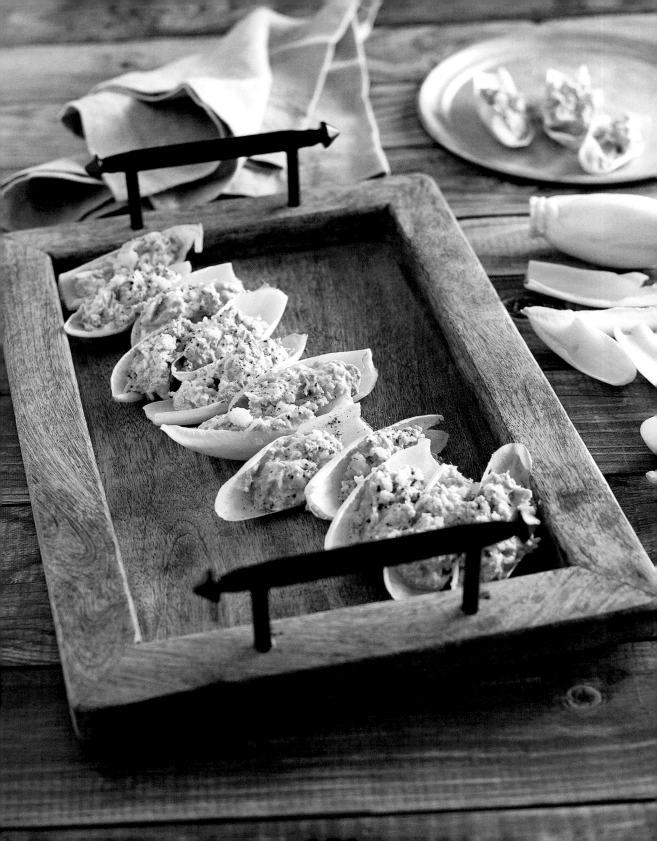

# KITCHEN SINK ENDIVE CUPS

*This recipe has a bit of every good fat and protein you can use in your kitchen on a daily basis.*

**Makes 4 fat bombs**

1 large hard-boiled egg, peeled
2 tablespoons canned tuna in olive oil, drained
2 tablespoons avocado pulp
1 teaspoon fresh lime juice
1 tablespoon keto-approved mayonnaise
⅛ teaspoon sea salt
⅛ teaspoon black pepper
4 Belgian endive leaves, washed and dried

**1** In a small food processor, mix all ingredients except endive until well blended.

**2** Scoop 1 tablespoon tuna mixture onto each endive cup.

**3** Serve immediately.

**Per Serving**
Calories: 71 | Fat: 5.7 g | Protein: 3.8 g | Sodium: 114 mg | Fiber: 0.7 g | Carbohydrates: 1.1 g | Net Carbohydrates: 0.4 g | Sugar: 0.2 g

# CURRIED EGG SALAD ENDIVE CUPS

*The delicate but complex flavor of curry blends wonderfully with eggs, giving the egg salad a slightly unusual but successful twist.*

**Makes 2 fat bombs**

1 large hard-boiled egg, peeled
1 teaspoon curry powder
1 tablespoon coconut oil
⅛ teaspoon sea salt
⅛ teaspoon black pepper
2 Belgian endive leaves, washed and dried

**1** In a small food processor, mix all ingredients except endive until well blended.

**2** Scoop 1 tablespoon egg salad mixture onto each endive cup.

**3** Serve immediately.

**Per Serving**
Calories: 100 | Fat: 8.7 g | Protein: 3.4 g | Sodium: 129 mg | Fiber: 0.7 g | Carbohydrates: 1.1 g | Net Carbohydrates: 0.4 g | Sugar: 0.3 g

# BEET CHIPS

*Beets have a lot of red pigment; that's why they're commonly used as a natural red dye. When peeling and slicing beets, you may want to use food-safe gloves to avoid staining your fingers.*

**Serves 6**

10 medium red beets
½ cup avocado oil
2 teaspoons sea salt
½ teaspoon granulated garlic

**1** Preheat oven to 350°F. Line a few baking sheets with parchment paper and set aside.

**2** Peel beets with a vegetable slicer and cut off ends. Carefully slice beets into rounds, about 3 mm thick, with a mandoline slicer or a sharp knife.

**3** Place sliced beets in a large bowl and add oil, salt, and granulated garlic. Toss to coat each slice. Set aside 20 minutes, allowing salt to pull out excess moisture.

**4** Drain excess liquid and arrange sliced beets in a single layer on prepared baking sheets. Bake 45 minutes or until crisp.

**5** Remove from oven and allow to cool. Store in an airtight container until ready to eat, up to 1 week.

### Benefits of Beets

The red pigments in beets, called betalains, help reduce chronic inflammation, which is associated with a host of health issues. Beets can also improve brain and digestive health, reduce blood pressure, and increase your body's oxygen use by up to 20 percent.

**Per Serving**
Calories: 113 | Fat: 5.9 g | Protein: 2.2 g | Sodium: 279 mg | Fiber: 3.9 g | Carbohydrates: 13.3 g | Net Carbohydrates: 9.4 g | Sugar: 9.2 g

# SMOKED SALMON AND AVOCADO ROLLUPS

*Super-quick and easy dairy-free fat bombs, these rollups make a great party food or an easy appetizer.*

**Makes 3 fat bombs**

½ medium avocado, peeled and pitted (about 3 ounces)
1 teaspoon fresh lemon juice
⅛ teaspoon sea salt
3 (1-ounce) slices smoked salmon (lox)

**1** In a small bowl, combine avocado, lemon juice, and salt; mash with a fork.

**2** Spread ⅓ avocado mixture evenly on top of each salmon slice. Roll slices into individual rolls and secure with a toothpick.

**3** Serve immediately.

**Per Serving**
Calories: 71 | Fat: 4.2 g | Protein: 5.6 g | Sodium: 568 mg | Fiber: 1.6 g | Carbohydrates: 2.1 g | Net Carbohydrates: 0.5 g | Sugar: 0.1 g

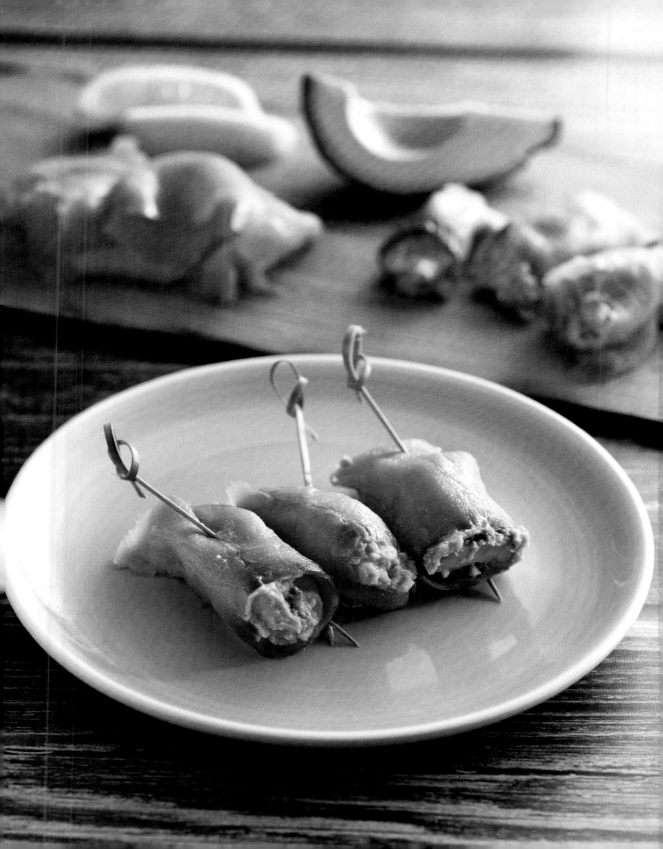

# MEDITERRANEAN ROLLUPS

*Olives and sun-dried tomatoes are the flavors of the Mediterranean Sea. From Italy to Greece, hot summer days include the tastes of ripe tomatoes and fresh olive oil and the scent of beautiful olive groves. This recipe will take you there!*

**Makes 2 fat bombs**

1 large egg
1 tablespoon extra-virgin olive oil
⅛ teaspoon sea salt
6 large kalamata olives, pitted
2 tablespoons sun-dried tomatoes in oil
⅛ teaspoon red chili flakes
⅛ teaspoon dried parsley

**1** In a small bowl, combine egg, olive oil, and salt and whisk until foamy.

**2** Heat a small nonstick skillet over high heat and pour in egg mixture, spreading evenly so it forms a thin, even layer.

**3** Once the first side is cooked, about 1 minute, flip frittata with the aid of a plate or a lid. Cook until golden on bottom, about 2 more minutes. Remove frittata to a plate.

**4** In a small food processor, mix olives, tomatoes, chili flakes, and parsley until well chopped and blended, about 30 seconds.

**5** Spread olive paste on top of frittata in an even layer.

**6** Roll frittata into a tight roll, cut into 2 pieces, and serve immediately.

**Per Serving**
Calories: 135 | Fat: 12.6 g | Protein: 3.5 g | Sodium: 323 mg | Fiber: 0.4 g | Carbohydrates: 1.8 g | Net Carbohydrates: 1.4 g | Sugar: 0.1 g

# DELI ROLLUPS

*Instead of purchasing prepared chive cream cheese, you can make your own by combining plain cream cheese with minced onions and dried chives.*

**Serves 2**

**8 (1-ounce) slices sugar-free deli ham**
**4 ounces (½ cup) chive cream cheese**
**1 cup chopped baby spinach**
**1 medium red bell pepper, seeded and sliced**

**1** Lay out each slice of ham flat. Spread 1 tablespoon cream cheese on each slice.

**2** Put 2 tablespoons chopped spinach on top of the cream cheese on each slice.

**3** Divide bell pepper into 8 equal portions and put portions on top of spinach.

**4** Roll up the ham and secure with a toothpick. Eat immediately or refrigerate until ready to serve.

**Per Serving**
Calories: 399 | Fat: 25.9 g | Protein: 23.2 g | Sodium: 1,515 mg | Fiber: 3.1 g | Carbohydrates: 10.8 g | Net Carbohydrates: 7.7 g | Sugar: 4.4 g

## Check Your Labels!

Many hams contain cane sugar, brown sugar, maple syrup, or honey. When choosing a ham, read your labels carefully and stay away from any that contain added sugars, which will up the carbohydrate content of this meal significantly.

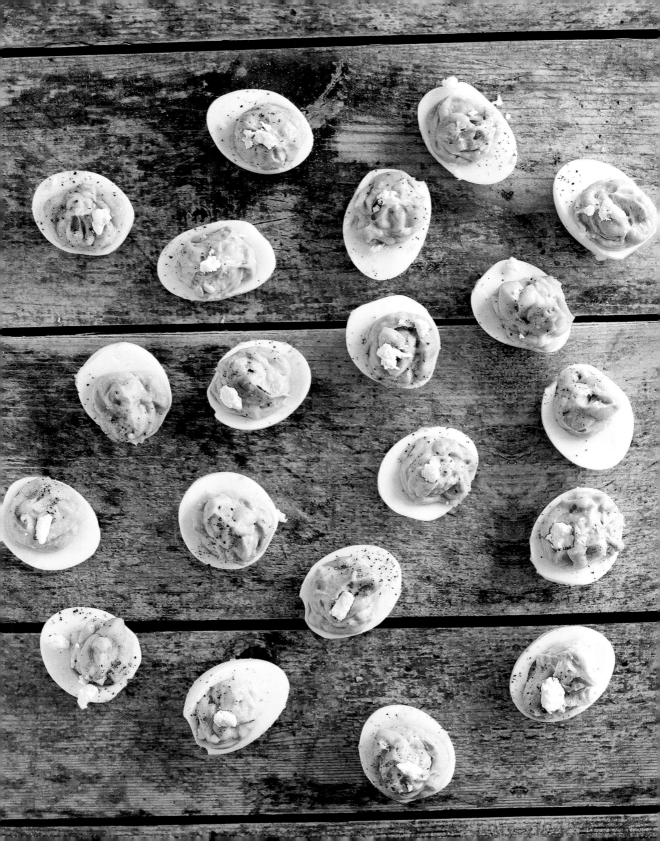

# GREEN DEVILED EGGS

*Adding avocado to traditional deviled eggs provides a healthy dose of monounsaturated fats and increases vitamin K, folate, vitamin C, and potassium content.*

**Serves 2**

4 large hard-boiled eggs

1 large avocado, peeled, pitted, and chopped

¼ cup keto-approved mayonnaise

1 teaspoon lime juice

1 tablespoon feta cheese

2 teaspoons light olive oil

⅛ teaspoon salt

¼ teaspoon black pepper

**1** Peel hard-boiled eggs and cut in half lengthwise. Scoop out yolks and place in a small bowl.

**2** Put remaining ingredients except pepper in bowl with egg yolks and mash with a fork until combined.

**3** Fill each egg white half with an equal amount of the yolk mixture. Sprinkle pepper on top.

**Per Serving**
Calories: 521 | Fat: 47.4 g | Protein: 14.6 g | Sodium: 466 mg | Fiber: 4.7 g | Carbohydrates: 7.6 g | Net Carbohydrates: 2.9 g | Sugar: 1.6 g

# RANCH DIP

*You can thin this dip out and use it as a dressing by adding some full-fat coconut milk or heavy cream, if you can tolerate dairy.*

**Serves 6**

1 cup keto-approved mayonnaise
½ cup plain Greek yogurt
1½ teaspoons dried chives
1½ teaspoons dried parsley
1½ teaspoons dried dill
¾ teaspoon granulated garlic
¾ teaspoon granulated onion
½ teaspoon salt
¼ teaspoon black pepper

**1** Combine all ingredients in a small bowl.

**2** Allow to sit in the refrigerator 30 minutes before serving.

**Per Serving**
Calories: 289 | Fat: 33.0 g | Protein: 1.9 g | Sodium: 401 mg | Fiber: 0.3 g | Carbohydrates: 1.7 g | Net Carbohydrates: 1.4 g | Sugar: 0.8 g

# TURKEY AVOCADO ROLLS

*Lemon pepper has a strong taste, so in this recipe, a little goes a long way. If you don't like the zing of lemon, try garlic pepper in place of the lemon pepper or just omit the spice blend completely.*

**Serves 4**

12 (1-ounce) slices turkey breast
12 (1-ounce) slices Swiss cheese
3 cups baby spinach
1 large avocado, peeled, pitted, and cut into 12 slices
¼ cup keto-approved mayonnaise
¼ teaspoon lemon pepper

**1** Lay out the slices of turkey breast flat and place a slice of Swiss cheese on top of each one.

**2** Top each slice with ¼ cup baby spinach and 3 slices avocado. Drizzle with 1 teaspoon mayonnaise.

**3** Sprinkle each "sandwich" with lemon pepper. Roll up sandwiches and secure with toothpicks. Serve immediately or refrigerate until ready to serve.

**Per Serving**
Calories: 569 | Fat: 40.2 g | Protein: 38.1 g | Sodium: 946 mg | Fiber: 2.8 g | Carbohydrates: 10.3 g | Net Carbohydrates: 7.5 g | Sugar: 4.1 g

## Check Your Spices

It may come as a surprise, but many commercial spices contain sugar or hydrogenated fats. Don't assume that an ingredient such as lemon pepper is free of carbohydrates until you check the label. If it contains sugar, ditch it and find one that doesn't. When it comes to herbs and spices, there are plenty of sugar-free options out there.

# BUFFALO CHICKEN FINGERS

*If you're making these Buffalo Chicken Fingers in advance, you can keep them crispier by adding the buffalo sauce right before you eat them instead of adding it to all the chicken fingers at once.*

**Serves 6**

2 cups almond flour

1 teaspoon salt

1 teaspoon black pepper

1 teaspoon dried parsley

2 large eggs

2 tablespoons full-fat canned coconut milk

2 pounds chicken tenders

1½ cups Frank's RedHot Buffalo sauce

**1** Preheat oven to 350°F.

**2** Combine almond flour, salt, pepper, and parsley in a medium bowl and set aside.

**3** Beat eggs and coconut milk together in a separate medium bowl.

**4** Dip each chicken tender into egg mixture and then coat completely with almond flour mixture. Arrange coated tenders in a single layer on a baking sheet.

**5** Bake 30 minutes, flipping once during cooking. Remove from oven and allow to cool 5 minutes.

**6** Place chicken tenders in a large bowl and add buffalo sauce. Toss to coat completely.

**Per Serving**
Calories: 320 | Fat: 17.1 g | Protein: 36.0 g | Sodium: 2,293 mg | Fiber: 3.1 g | Carbohydrates: 6.5 g | Net Carbohydrates: 3.4 g | Sugar: 1.1 g

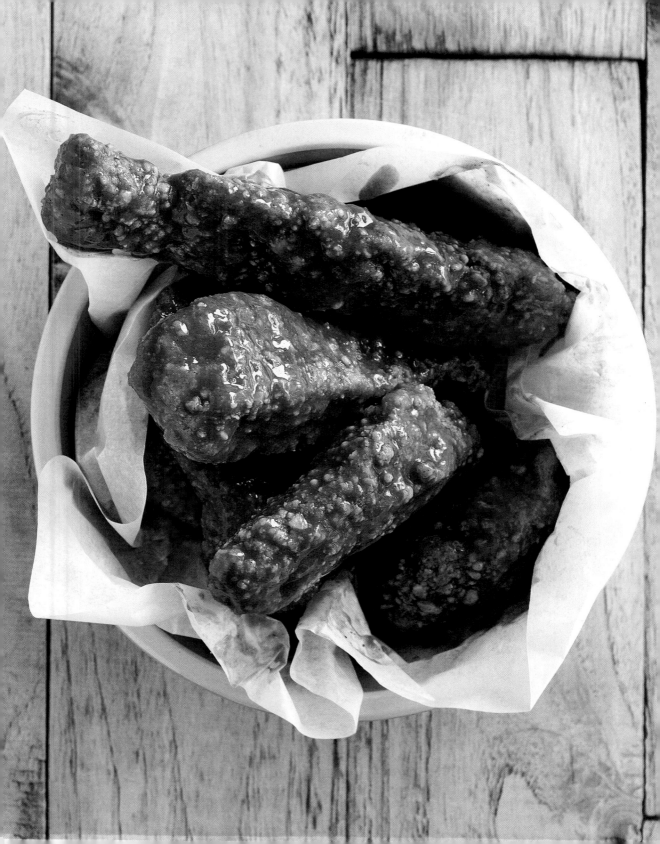

# BACON OLIVE SPREAD

*Bacon and olive are complementary salty flavors that pair well with cream cheese. This spread is great served on celery sticks or cucumber slices.*

**Serves 4**

4 slices no-sugar-added bacon
1 (8-ounce) package cream cheese, softened to room temperature
2 tablespoons olive oil mayonnaise
1 tablespoon freshly squeezed lemon juice
24 Spanish olives, sliced

**1** Cook bacon in a large skillet over medium heat until crisp, 5 minutes per side. Drain on paper towel.

**2** In a medium mixing bowl, beat softened cream cheese with a hand mixer until smooth.

**3** Add mayonnaise and lemon juice and mix on medium speed until combined.

**4** Crumble bacon into bowl followed by sliced olives. Fold into cream cheese mixture by hand with a rubber spatula.

**5** Can be served immediately or cooled in refrigerator to enjoy cold.

**Per Serving**
Calories: 287 | Fat: 24.0 g | Protein: 7.4 g | Sodium: 588 mg | Fiber: 0.6 g | Carbohydrates: 5.0 g | Net Carbohydrates: 4.4 g | Sugar: 2.1 g

# CHORIZO-STUFFED JALAPEÑOS

*There is perhaps no better pairing than chorizo with spicy peppers baked into a delicious creamy mound of cheese. The addition of bacon is truly the icing on the cake.*

**Makes 6 fat bombs**

1 tablespoon olive oil

¼ medium yellow onion, peeled and minced

6 ounces pork chorizo sausage

4 ounces (½ cup) cream cheese, softened to room temperature

3 medium jalapeño peppers, seeded and sliced in half

3 slices no-sugar-added bacon, sliced in half horizontally

**1** Preheat oven to 375°F.

**2** Add olive oil to a medium skillet over medium heat and sweat onions 2 minutes. Add chorizo to skillet and cook another 3–5 minutes. Drain mixture.

**3** In medium mixing bowl, whip cream cheese with hand mixer until softened. Fold in sausage and onion mixture with a spatula.

**4** Stuff each pepper half with cream cheese mixture.

**5** Wrap 1 bacon slice around each stuffed pepper in a spiral motion, covering the cream cheese mixture underneath.

**6** Bake 10–15 minutes or until bacon becomes crispy and cream cheese mixture underneath bubbles through and turns slightly brown. Serve warm.

**Per Serving**
Calories: 219 | Fat: 18.0 g | Protein: 8.9 g | Sodium: 447 mg | Fiber: 0.3 g | Carbohydrates: 2.2 g | Net Carbohydrates: 1.9 g | Sugar: 1.1 g

## Why Do Americans Love Jalapeño Poppers?

Although their origin is a bit fuzzy, poppers were speculated to be an American spin-off of the Mexican classic chiles rellenos. Nobody can seem to pinpoint who coined the term *poppers* and decided to batter dip, freeze, and commercialize them in the 1980s, but they have been a popular restaurant staple in California since at least the 1960s.

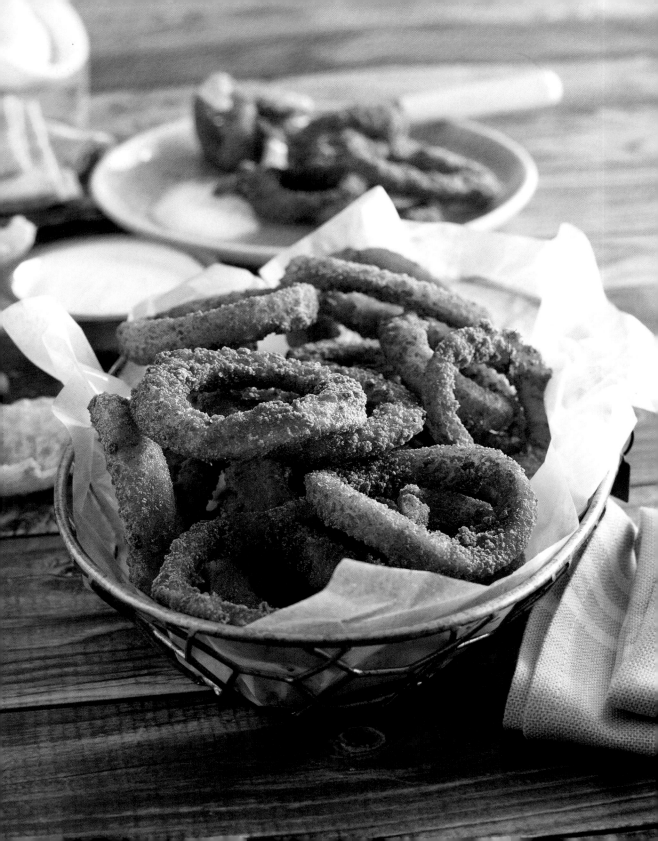

# ONION RINGS

*Onion rings are a comfort food staple, but traditional onion rings are out on a ketogenic diet. This recipe uses low-carb pork rinds in place of breading so you can enjoy this fan favorite with significantly fewer carbohydrates. Serve these with Ranch Dip (see recipe in this chapter).*

**Serves 6**

2 medium white onions, peeled and sliced into ½" rings
4 large eggs
⅓ cup full-fat canned coconut milk
1 cup pork rinds, crushed
¾ cup grated Parmesan cheese
1 cup coconut flour

**1** Preheat oven to 425°F.

**2** Break onion rings apart, removing smaller inside pieces and reserving only the rings.

**3** Whisk together eggs and coconut milk in a medium bowl. Combine crushed pork rinds and Parmesan cheese in a separate medium bowl. Place coconut flour in a third medium bowl.

**4** Dip each onion ring in coconut flour, then egg wash, then pork rind mixture. Repeat this process to double coat onion rings.

**5** Line onion rings on a baking rack and bake 15–20 minutes or until onion rings are golden and crispy.

**Per Serving**
Calories: 246 | Fat: 12.6 g | Protein: 16.8 g | Sodium: 421 mg | Fiber: 6.0 g | Carbohydrates: 14.9 g | Net Carbohydrates: 8.9 g | Sugar: 4.9 g

# CHICKEN SKIN CRISPS ALFREDO

*Alfredo sauce must be one of the most well-loved sauces for both chicken and noodles. Here you can get all the flavor of Alfredo sauce without any of the carbs usually involved!*

**Makes 6 fat bombs**

Skin from 3 large chicken thighs
2 tablespoons ricotta cheese
2 tablespoons cream cheese
1 tablespoon grated Parmesan cheese
¼ clove garlic, minced
¼ teaspoon ground white pepper

**1** Preheat oven to 350°F. On a cookie sheet lined with parchment paper, lay out skins as flat as possible.

**2** Bake 12–15 minutes until skins turn light brown and crispy, being careful not to burn them.

**3** Remove skins from cookie sheet and place on a paper towel to cool.

**4** In a small bowl, add cheeses, garlic, and pepper. Mix with a fork until well blended.

**5** Cut each crispy chicken skin in 2 pieces.

**6** Place 1 tablespoon cheese mix on each chicken crisp and serve immediately.

### Chicken Skin Crisps

You can either buy chicken thighs and remove the skin to make your chicken skin crisps, or you can ask your local butcher or farmer from the farmers' market to sell you just chicken skin. You will be surprised; chicken skin is not so hard to find, and it will make superb crisps to use instead of crackers.

**Per Serving**
Calories: 94 | Fat: 7.9 g | Protein: 3.5 g | Sodium: 48 mg | Fiber: 0.0 g | Carbohydrates: 0.6 g | Net Carbohydrates: 0.6 g | Sugar: 0.2 g

# CHEESY MUFFIN PROSCIUTTO CUP

*Salty prosciutto, creamy melted cheeses, and a nourishing egg—sounds like a perfect combination.*

**Makes 1 fat bomb**

**1 slice prosciutto (about ½ ounce)**
**1 medium egg yolk**
**3 tablespoons diced Brie**
**2 tablespoons diced mozzarella cheese**
**3 tablespoons grated Parmesan cheese**

**1** Preheat oven to 350°F. Take out a muffin tin with wells about 2½" wide and 1½" deep.

**2** Fold prosciutto slice in half so it becomes almost square. Place it in muffin tin well to line it completely.

**3** Place egg yolk into prosciutto cup.

**4** Add cheeses on top of egg yolk gently without breaking it.

**5** Bake about 12 minutes until yolk is cooked and warm but still runny.

**6** Let cool 10 minutes before removing from muffin tin.

**Per Serving**
Calories: 290 | Fat: 21.0 g | Protein: 18.7 g | Sodium: 590 mg | Fiber: 0.0 g | Carbohydrates: 3.5 g | Net Carbohydrates: 3.5 g | Sugar: 0.4 g

# BACON JALAPEÑO BALLS

*Enjoy a little kick of fire in these Mexican-flavored fat bombs.*

**Makes 6 fat bombs**

**5 slices no-sugar-added bacon, cooked, fat reserved**

**¼ cup plus 2 tablespoons (3 ounces) cream cheese**

**2 tablespoons reserved bacon fat**

**1 teaspoon seeded and finely chopped jalapeño pepper**

**1 tablespoon finely chopped cilantro**

**1** On a cutting board, chop bacon into small crumbs.

**2** In a small bowl, combine cream cheese, bacon fat, jalapeño, and cilantro; mix well with a fork.

**3** Form mixture into 6 balls.

**4** Place bacon crumbles on a medium plate and roll individual balls through to coat evenly.

**5** Serve immediately or refrigerate up to 3 days.

**Per Serving**
Calories: 132 | Fat: 11.5 g | Protein: 4.1 g | Sodium: 219 mg | Fiber: 0.1 g | Carbohydrates: 0.9 g | Net Carbohydrates: 0.8 g | Sugar: 0.6 g

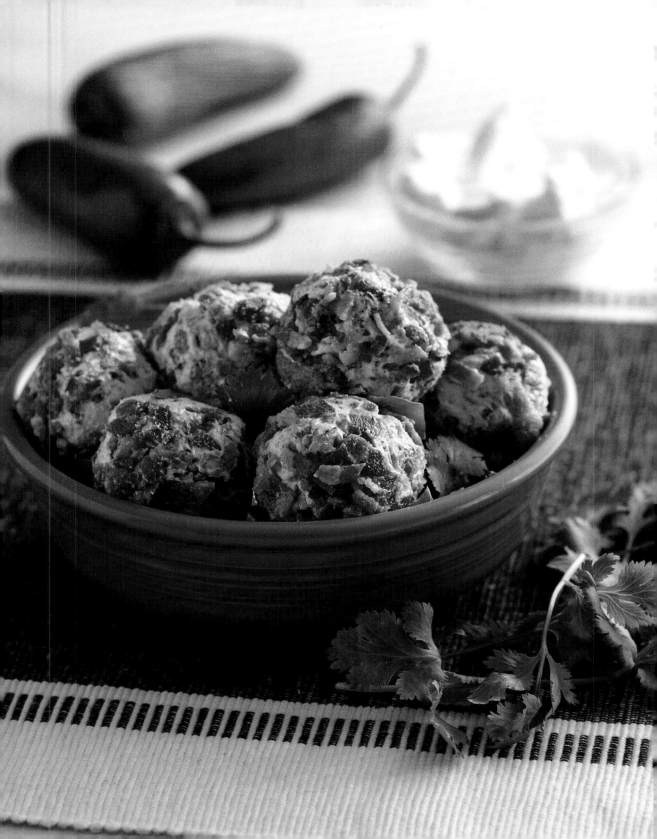

# AVOCADO, MACADAMIA, AND PROSCIUTTO BALLS

*The subtle, smooth flavors of avocado and macadamia nuts make a perfect counterpoint for salty prosciutto and spicy pepper.*

**Makes 6 fat bombs**

½ cup macadamia nuts
½ large avocado, peeled and pitted (about 4 ounces pulp)
1 ounce cooked prosciutto, crumbled
¼ teaspoon black pepper

**1** In a small food processor, pulse macadamia nuts until evenly crumbled. Divide in half.

**2** In a small bowl, combine avocado, half the macadamia nuts, prosciutto crumbles, and pepper and mix well with a fork.

**3** Form mixture into 6 balls.

**4** Place remaining crumbled macadamia nuts on a medium plate and roll individual balls through to coat evenly.

**5** Serve immediately.

**Per Serving**
Calories: 113 | Fat: 10.7 g | Protein: 2.1 g | Sodium: 20 mg | Fiber: 1.8 g | Carbohydrates: 2.7 g | Net Carbohydrates: 0.9 g | Sugar: 0.5 g

# PEPPERONI CHIPS

*Make sure to thoroughly blot away the excess grease in this recipe. If you don't, you'll end up with soggy chips instead of crispy ones.*

**Serves 4**

**24 slices sugar-free pepperoni**

**1** Preheat oven to 425°F.

**2** Line a baking sheet with parchment paper and lay out pepperoni slices in a single layer.

**3** Bake 10 minutes and then remove from oven and use a paper towel to blot away excess grease. Return to the oven 5 more minutes or until pepperoni is crispy.

**Per Serving**
Calories: 59 | Fat: 4.3 g | Protein: 2.8 g | Sodium: 211 mg | Fiber: 0.0 g | Carbohydrates: 0.0 g | Net Carbohydrates: 0.0 g | Sugar: 0.0 g

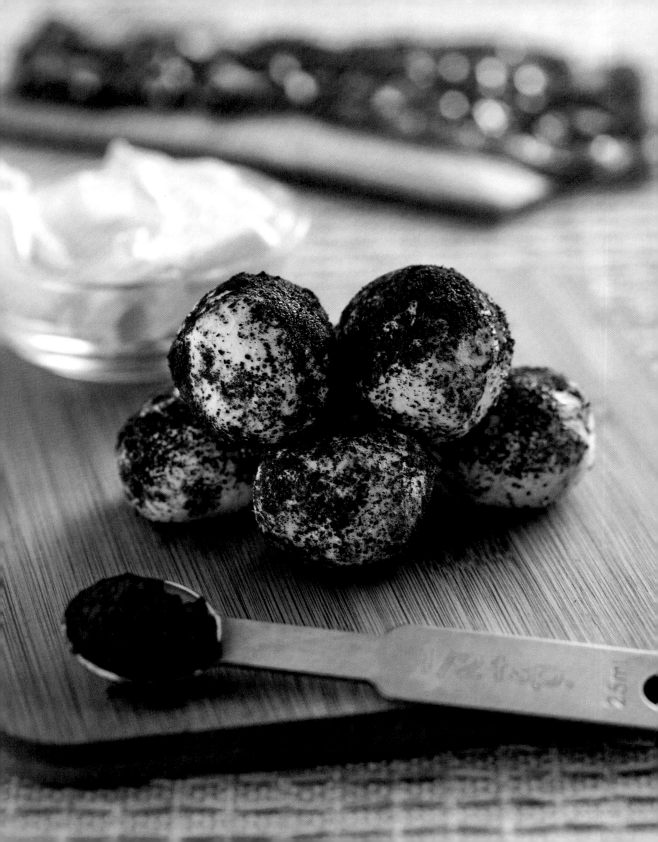

# BARBECUE BALLS

*An easy way to get your barbecue fix— and your fat too. You will be surprised how much these fat bombs taste like barbecue sauce.*

**Makes 6 fat bombs**

4 ounces (½ cup) cream cheese
4 tablespoons bacon fat
½ teaspoon smoke flavor
2 drops stevia glycerite
⅛ teaspoon apple cider vinegar
1 tablespoon sweet smoked chili powder

**1** In a small food processor, process all ingredients except chili powder until they form a smooth cream, about 30 seconds.

**2** Scrape mixture and transfer into a small bowl, then refrigerate 2 hours.

**3** Form into 6 balls with the aid of a spoon.

**4** Sprinkle balls with chili powder, rolling around to coat all sides.

**5** Serve immediately or refrigerate up to 3 days.

**Per Serving**
Calories: 146 | Fat: 14.0 g | Protein: 1.3 g | Sodium: 121 mg | Fiber: 0.5 g | Carbohydrates: 1.5 g | Net Carbohydrates: 1.0 g | Sugar: 0.7 g

# GOAT CHEESE AND HERBS PANNA COTTA

*Herbed goat cheese is a very popular item in fancy cheese stores. Now you can replicate that fancy flavor with the right amount of good fat for your keto diet.*

**Makes 6 fat bombs**

1½ cups heavy whipping cream
¾ cup full-fat sour cream
6 ounces soft goat cheese
1 teaspoon Herbes de Provence
2 teaspoons powdered unflavored gelatin
1 teaspoon sea salt

**1** In a small saucepan over medium heat, combine heavy cream, sour cream, goat cheese, and Herbes de Provence, stirring until cheese melts.

**2** Whisk in gelatin and salt until completely incorporated. Simmer over very low heat about 5 minutes, stirring constantly.

**3** Pour mixture evenly into 6 small glasses or ramekins. Refrigerate until set, at least 6 hours or overnight.

**4** Serve in glass or ramekin or invert over a small plate after dipping glass or ramekin into hot water a few seconds.

**Per Serving**
Calories: 371 | Fat: 33.9 g | Protein: 9.9 g | Sodium: 418 mg | Fiber: 0.0 g | Carbohydrates: 2.5 g | Net Carbohydrates: 2.5 g | Sugar: 2.5 g

# BACON AND SCALLION BITES

*Not all cheesecakes are sweet. With bacon and scallions in the mix, this version makes an excellent savory appetizer or midday snack.*

**Makes 6 fat bombs**

⅓ cup almond meal

1 tablespoon unsalted butter, melted

1 (8-ounce) package cream cheese, softened to room temperature

1 tablespoon bacon grease

1 large egg

4 slices no-sugar-added bacon, cooked, cooled, and crumbled into bits

1 large green onion, tops only, thinly sliced

1 clove garlic, minced

⅛ teaspoon black pepper

## Savor the Savory Flavor

Perhaps not as popular, but certainly as delicious, the savory cheesecake makes for an excellent treat. Most savory cakes served in restaurants include flavor combinations such as garlic and Parmesan, bacon and chive, and prosciutto and olive.

**1** Preheat oven to 325°F.

**2** In a small mixing bowl, combine almond meal and butter.

**3** Line 6 cups of a standard-sized muffin tin with cupcake liners. Equally divide almond meal mixture among cups and press into the bottom gently with the back of a teaspoon. Bake in oven 10 minutes, then remove.

**4** While the crust is baking, thoroughly combine cream cheese and bacon grease in a medium mixing bowl with a hand mixer. Add egg and blend until combined.

**5** Fold bacon, onion, garlic, and pepper into cream cheese mixture with a spatula.

**6** Divide mixture among cups, return to oven, and bake another 30–35 minutes until cheese sets. Edges may be slightly browned. To test doneness, insert toothpick into center. If it comes out clean, cheesecake is done.

**7** Let cool 5 minutes and serve.

**Per Serving**
Calories: 249 | Fat: 21.3 g | Protein: 7.3 g | Sodium: 282 mg | Fiber: 0.7 g | Carbohydrates: 3.3 g | Net Carbohydrates: 2.6 g | Sugar: 1.5 g

# PIZZA BALLS

*This recipe takes the ultimate Italian dish and magically transforms it into a fat bomb. Whenever the urge for pizza hits you, reach for this instead.*

**Makes 6 fat bombs**

¼ cup (2 ounces) fresh mozzarella cheese

2 ounces (¼ cup) cream cheese

1 tablespoon olive oil

1 teaspoon tomato paste

6 large kalamata olives, pitted

12 fresh basil leaves

**1** In a small food processor, process all ingredients except basil until they form a smooth cream, about 30 seconds.

**2** Form mixture into 6 balls with the aid of a spoon.

**3** Place 1 basil leaf on top and bottom of each ball and secure with a toothpick.

**4** Serve immediately or refrigerate up to 3 days.

**Per Serving**
Calories: 76 | Fat: 7.0 g | Protein: 1.7 g | Sodium: 122 mg | Fiber: 0.1 g | Carbohydrates: 0.7 g | Net Carbohydrates: 0.6 g | Sugar: 0.5 g

# PORCINI MUSHROOM PANNA COTTA

*This recipe will make a great impression on the guests at a dinner party...and they will never know you are just serving a fat bomb.*

**Makes 6 fat bombs**

¼ cup (2 ounces) dried porcini mushrooms
1 cup hot water
1 teaspoon powdered unflavored gelatin
1 tablespoon unsalted butter
1 cup heavy cream
1 tablespoon coconut aminos
3 tablespoons grated Parmesan cheese

**1** Soak porcini mushrooms in hot water about 30 minutes to rehydrate.

**2** Drain mushrooms, reserving the soaking water. Squeeze out excess water from mushrooms, then chop finely.

**3** Place 3 tablespoons soaking water in a glass. Sprinkle gelatin in soaking water and let stand about 5 minutes.

**4** In a small nonstick skillet over high heat, melt butter, then add mushrooms and sauté about 3 minutes, stirring.

**5** Add soaking water with gelatin, cream, coconut aminos, and Parmesan cheese; stir and bring to a boil, about 1 minute.

**6** Remove from heat.

**7** Pour mixture evenly into 6 small glasses or ramekins. Refrigerate until set, at least 6 hours or overnight.

**8** Serve in glass or ramekin or invert over a small plate after dipping glass or ramekin into hot water a few seconds.

### Skip the Soy

Coconut aminos sauce is a soy-free seasoning made from the sap of coconut blossoms that you can use in place of soy sauce in any of your recipes. There is absolutely no coconut flavor—it tastes just like soy sauce—but unlike soy sauce, which is highly processed and most likely contains GMOs, coconut aminos are GMO-free and contain seventeen amino acids, vitamins, and minerals.

**Per Serving**
Calories: 198 | Fat: 16.4 g | Protein: 3.5 g | Sodium: 120 mg | Fiber: 1.1 g | Carbohydrates: 9.1 g | Net Carbohydrates: 8.0 g | Sugar: 1.3 g

# KALAMATA OLIVE AND FETA BALLS

*This recipe brings you the flavors of Greece on a warm sunny day by the Mediterranean Sea.*

**Makes 6 fat bombs**

2 ounces (¼ cup) cream cheese
¼ cup (2 ounces) feta cheese
12 large kalamata olives, pitted
⅛ teaspoon finely chopped fresh thyme
⅛ teaspoon fresh lemon zest

**1** In a small food processor, process all ingredients until they form a coarse dough, about 30 seconds.

**2** Scrape mixture and transfer to a small bowl, then refrigerate 2 hours.

**3** Form into 6 balls with the aid of a spoon.

**4** Serve immediately or refrigerate up to 3 days.

**Per Serving**
Calories: 67 | Fat: 6.1 g | Protein: 1.5 g | Sodium: 207 mg | Fiber: 0.0 g | Carbohydrates: 0.7 g | Net Carbohydrates: 0.7 g | Sugar: 0.6 g

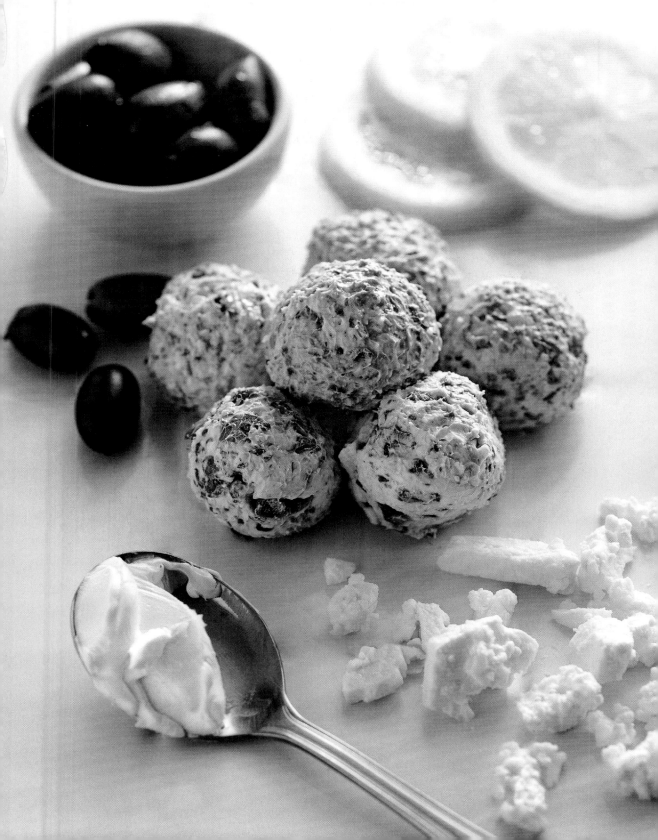

# STUFFED BABY BELLA MUSHROOM CAPS

*Mushrooms make an excellent holder for meat-based fat bombs. These bombs use a hearty and earthy-tasting mushroom filled with the proper proportion of tangy cheese and savory sausage.*

**Makes 8 fat bombs**

1 tablespoon olive oil

8 baby bella mushrooms, cleaned and stems removed

¼ teaspoon salt

4 ounces pork breakfast sausage at room temperature

4 tablespoons chopped fresh parsley

½ cup shredded Parmesan cheese

**1** Preheat oven to 350°F.

**2** Rub olive oil on mushroom tops and sprinkle lightly with salt.

**3** Mix sausage, parsley, and Parmesan cheese in a small mixing bowl.

**4** Stuff each mushroom cap until mixture forms a nice cap slightly above the mushroom ribbing.

**5** Bake on a cookie sheet about 20 minutes until sausage becomes browned and cheese browns slightly. Serve warm.

**Per Serving**
Calories: 86 | Fat: 6.2 g | Protein: 4.5 g | Sodium: 251 mg | Fiber: 0.2 g | Carbohydrates: 2.3 g | Net Carbohydrates: 2.1 g | Sugar: 0.5 g

# BRIE HAZELNUT BALLS

*This is another super-easy fat-bomb recipe bursting with delicious flavor. The warm notes of toasted hazelnuts and the fresh flavor of thyme really brighten the soft flavor of Brie.*

**Makes 6 fat bombs**

½ cup (4 ounces) Brie
¼ cup toasted hazelnuts
⅛ teaspoon finely chopped fresh thyme

**1** In a small food processor, process all ingredients until they form a coarse dough, about 30 seconds.

**2** Scrape mixture, transfer to a small bowl, and refrigerate 2 hours.

**3** Form into 6 balls with the aid of a spoon.

**4** Serve immediately or refrigerate up to 3 days.

**Per Serving**
Calories: 98 | Fat: 8.2 g | Protein: 4.8 g | Sodium: 118 mg | Fiber: 0.6 g | Carbohydrates: 1.0 g | Net Carbohydrates: 0.4 g | Sugar: 0.3 g

# CURRIED TUNA BALLS

*Just a touch of spice gives this recipe a different twist on the usual fat bomb. It's enough to keep your taste buds entertained and satisfied.*

**Makes 6 fat bombs**

¼ cup plus 2 tablespoons (3 ounces) tuna in oil, drained
2 ounces (¼ cup) cream cheese
¼ teaspoon curry powder, divided
2 tablespoons crumbled macadamia nuts

**1** In a small food processor, process tuna, cream cheese, and half the curry powder until they form a smooth cream, about 30 seconds.

**2** Form mixture into 6 balls.

**3** Place crumbled macadamia nuts and remaining curry powder on a medium plate and roll individual balls through to coat evenly.

**4** Serve immediately or refrigerate up to 3 days.

**Per Serving**
Calories: 79 | Fat: 5.9 g | Protein: 4.6 g | Sodium: 91 mg | Fiber: 0.3 g | Carbohydrates: 0.8 g | Net Carbohydrates: 0.5 g | Sugar: 0.4 g

## Mercury Concerns

If you're concerned about the mercury in tuna, keep in mind that adults can safely eat 18–24 ounces of tuna per month without a significant amount of mercury getting into their systems. If you'd like, swap out the tuna for canned salmon. Canned salmon is higher in omega-3 fatty acids and contains lower levels of mercury.

# FOR THE LOVE OF PORK BOMBS

*Any day with bacon is a great day. Add liverwurst, pistachios, and cream cheese, and the flavors become a symphony of perfect pork cuisine for any true bacon lover!*

**Makes 12 fat bombs**

8 slices no-sugar-added bacon
8 ounces Braunschweiger at room temperature
¼ cup chopped pistachios
6 ounces (¾ cup) cream cheese, softened to room temperature
1 teaspoon Dijon mustard

## Is Braunschweiger the Same As Liverwurst?

While the ingredients in both sausages are similar (pork and pork liver), many times Braunschweiger also contains bacon. Braunschweiger is generally soft and spreadable, whereas liverwurst is firmer and better for slicing.

**1** Cook bacon in a medium skillet over medium heat until crisp, 5 minutes per side. Drain on paper towels and let cool. Once cooled, crumble into bacon-bit-sized pieces.

**2** Place Braunschweiger with pistachios in a small food processor and pulse until just combined.

**3** In a small mixing bowl, use a hand blender to whip cream cheese and Dijon mustard until combined and fluffy.

**4** Divide meat mixture into 12 equal servings. Roll into balls and cover in a thin layer of cream cheese mixture.

**5** Chill at least 1 hour. When ready to serve, place bacon bits on a medium plate, roll balls through to coat evenly, and enjoy.

**6** Fat bombs can be refrigerated in an airtight container up to 4 days.

**Per Serving**
Calories: 161 | Fat: 12.6 g | Protein: 6.8 g | Sodium: 375 mg | Fiber: 0.3 g | Carbohydrates: 2.1 g | Net Carbohydrates: 1.8 g | Sugar: 0.7 g

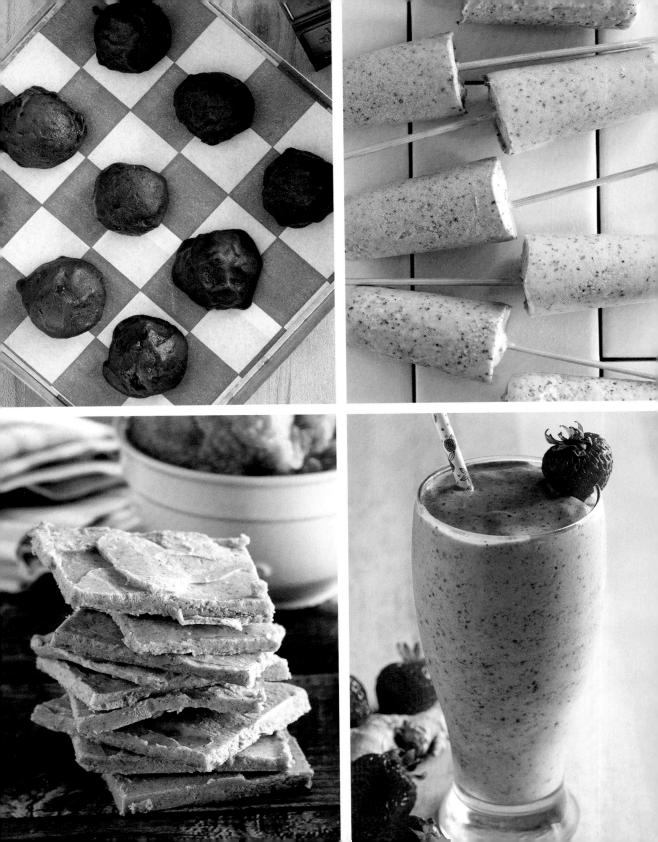

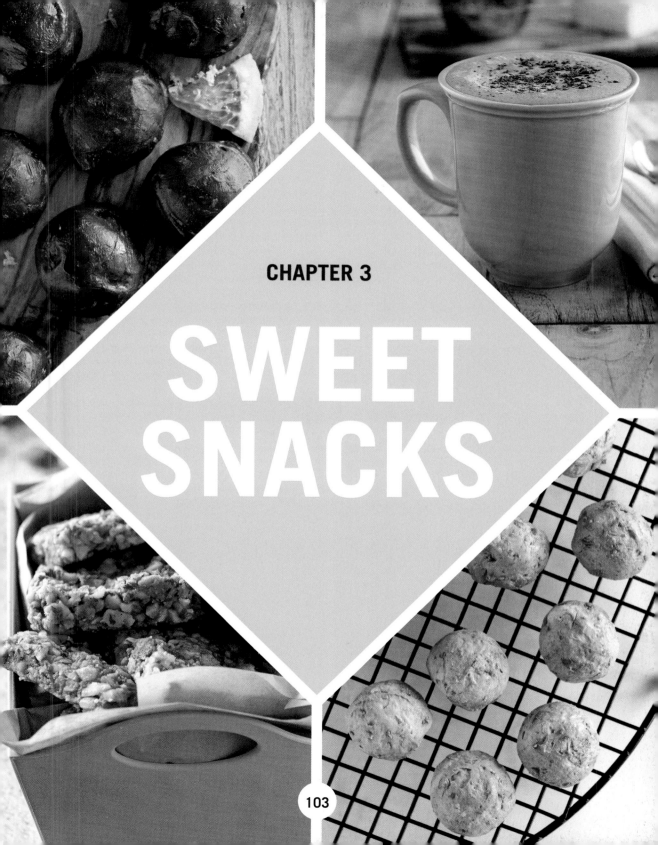

CHAPTER 3

# SWEET SNACKS

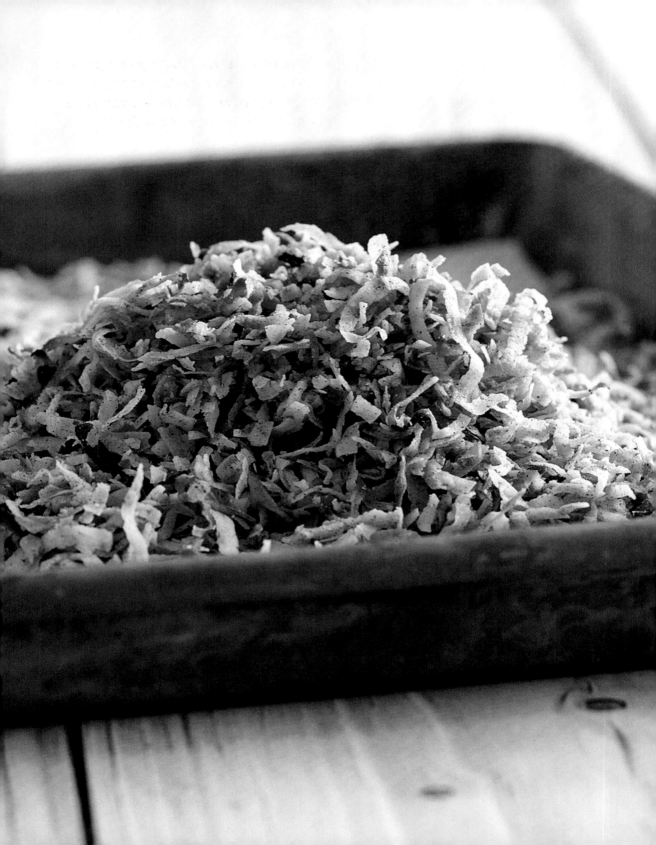

# PUMPKIN PIE COCONUT CRISPS

*The possibilities for this recipe are endless. You can experiment with any combination of spices you want. Make the crisps sweet or savory or a combination of both.*

**Serves 4**

**2 tablespoons coconut oil**
**½ teaspoon vanilla extract**
**½ teaspoon pumpkin pie spice**
**1 tablespoon granulated erythritol**
**2 cups unsweetened coconut flakes**
**⅛ teaspoon salt**

**1** Preheat oven to 350°F.

**2** Put coconut oil in a medium microwave-safe bowl and microwave until melted, about 20 seconds. Add vanilla extract, pumpkin pie spice, and granulated erythritol to coconut oil and stir until combined.

**3** Place coconut flakes in a medium bowl, pour coconut oil mixture over them, and toss to coat. Spread out in a single layer on a cookie sheet and sprinkle with salt.

**4** Bake 5 minutes or until coconut is crispy.

**Per Serving**
Calories: 327 | Fat: 30.4 g | Protein: 2.7 g | Sodium: 72 mg | Fiber: 8.0 g | Carbohydrates: 14.6 g | Net Carbohydrates: 2.8 g | Sugar Alcohols: 3.8 g | Sugar: 2.8 g

### Cuckoo for Coconuts

Coconuts are rich in a specific type of fat called medium-chain triglycerides (MCTs). Instead of circulating through the blood like other fats, MCTs go straight to the liver where they're burned for energy. Because your body doesn't store MCTs, eating them can help boost weight loss.

# ALMOND BUTTER BARK

*This recipe calls for almond butter, but you can make it with your favorite nut or seed butter, and the results will still be fantastic.*

**Serves 6**

½ cup no-sugar-added creamy almond butter

½ cup plus 1 teaspoon coconut oil, divided

2 teaspoons vanilla extract

6 drops liquid stevia

1 cup chopped walnuts

½ cup stevia-sweetened chocolate chips

**1** Line a rimmed baking sheet with parchment paper.

**2** Combine almond butter and ½ cup coconut oil in a small saucepan over medium-low heat. Stir until melted and combined. Stir in vanilla extract, stevia, and walnuts.

**3** Pour mixture onto lined baking sheet and spread out evenly.

**4** Combine chocolate chips and 1 teaspoon coconut oil in a small saucepan over low heat and stir to combine. Once melted, drizzle over almond butter mixture.

**5** Put baking sheet in freezer and freeze 30 minutes or until hardened. Remove from freezer and break into chunks.

**6** Store in an airtight container in the refrigerator or freezer until ready to eat.

## Sweetened with Stevia

If you're unable to find stevia-sweetened chocolate chips for this recipe, you can either leave the chocolate drizzle out completely or make your own. To make your own, combine unsweetened baking chocolate with coconut oil and add a drop or two of liquid stevia until you reach your desired sweetness level.

**Per Serving**
Calories: 473 | Fat: 45.6 g | Protein: 8.0 g | Sodium: 0 mg | Fiber: 7.5 g | Carbohydrates: 17.6 g | Net Carbohydrates: 7.1 g | Sugar Alcohols: 3.0 g | Sugar: 0.7 g

# CASHEW BUTTER BARS

*These Cashew Butter Bars will melt and fall apart if left at room temperature, so make sure to store them in the refrigerator or freezer.*

**Serves 6**

1½ cups no-sugar-added creamy cashew butter
½ cup granulated erythritol
¼ cup coconut flour
⅓ cup coconut oil, melted
¼ teaspoon salt

**1** Combine all ingredients in a medium mixing bowl and beat with a handheld mixer until fully incorporated.

**2** Transfer mixture to an 8" × 8" pan lined with parchment paper. Press evenly into pan.

**3** Refrigerate 2 hours or until bars set. Cut into 12 bars and store in an airtight container in the refrigerator until ready to eat, up to 2 weeks.

**Per Serving**
Calories: 500 | Fat: 42.1 g | Protein: 12.2 g | Sodium: 109 mg | Fiber: 3.0 g | Carbohydrates: 40.6 g | Net Carbohydrates: 17.6 g | Sugar Alcohols: 20.0 g | Sugar: 1.0 g

### An Easy Keto Snack

No-bake bars and balls like these Cashew Butter Bars make a great keto snack because they're quick and easy to make, and they're portable. You can save yourself some time in the future by doubling or tripling the batch and storing them in the freezer up to 3 months.

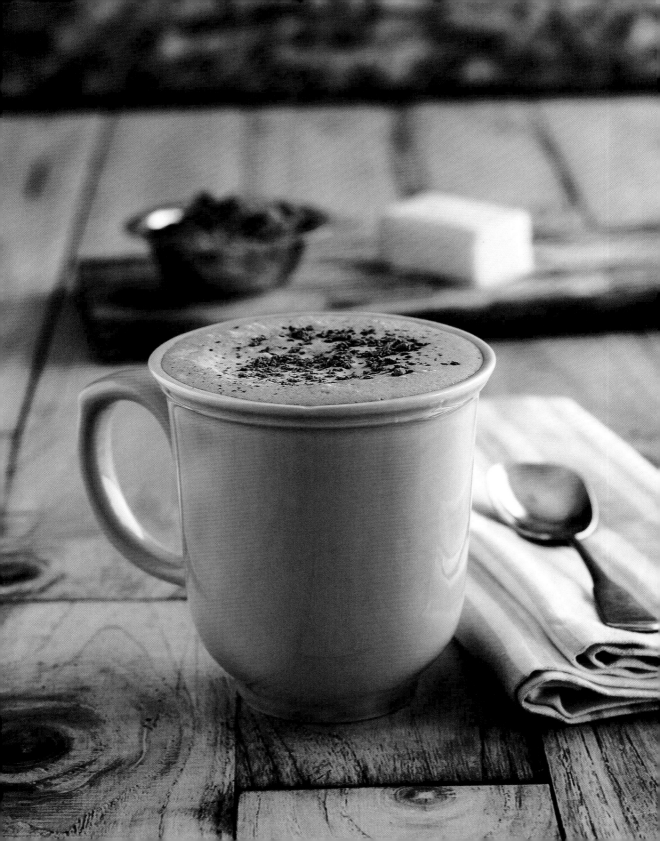

# BUTTER HOT CHOCOLATE

*This Butter Hot Chocolate is the perfect pick-me-up for that afternoon slump or after-dinner keto treat. It's easy to whip up with ingredients that you likely already have on hand.*

**Serves 1**

1 cup full-fat canned coconut milk
2 tablespoons unsalted grass-fed butter
2 teaspoons coconut oil
2 tablespoons unsweetened raw cacao powder
½ teaspoon vanilla extract
1 teaspoon granulated erythritol

**1** Add coconut milk to a small saucepan and bring to a simmer over medium heat. Once coconut milk reaches your desired temperature, transfer to a blender and add remaining ingredients.

**2** Blend until smooth and frothy.

**3** Pour into a mug and enjoy immediately.

**Per Serving**
Calories: 788 | Fat: 78.8 g | Protein: 6.6 g | Sodium: 99 mg | Fiber: 2.0 g | Carbohydrates: 17.6 g | Net Carbohydrates: 10.6 g | Sugar Alcohols: 5.0 g | Sugar: 0.3 g

## Give It a Kick

If you want a little extra caffeine boost, you can replace the coconut milk in this recipe with some brewed coffee—or use a combination of both.

# BLUEBERRY GRANOLA

*You can use fresh or frozen blueberries for this recipe, but stay away from dried blueberries. Because the water has been removed from dried blueberries, their sugar content is higher (and they're easier to overeat), and it will alter the carbohydrate content of this recipe.*

**Serves 6**

1 cup crushed raw almonds
½ cup crushed raw walnuts
½ cup crushed raw cashews
½ cup unsweetened shredded coconut
½ cup no-sugar-added cashew butter
¼ cup ground flaxseeds
4 tablespoons coconut oil, melted
1 cup frozen wild blueberries

**Go Wild**

Wild blueberries are richer in the purple pigment that gives them their color than conventional blueberries. This purple pigment is associated with the major health benefits of blueberries. If you can't find wild blueberries, you can use conventional blueberries in their place.

**1** Preheat oven to 200°F. Line a baking sheet with parchment paper.

**2** Combine all ingredients in a medium bowl and toss to combine. Spread out on baking sheet.

**3** Bake 4 hours or until golden and crispy. Remove from oven and allow to cool.

**4** Transfer to an airtight container and store in the refrigerator until ready to eat.

**Per Serving**
Calories: 409 | Fat: 34.5 g | Protein: 8.8 g | Sodium: 6 mg | Fiber: 5.2 g | Carbohydrates: 17.5 g | Net Carbohydrates: 12.3 g | Sugar: 3.6 g

# SNICKERDOODLE ROASTED NUTS

*When making these roasted nuts, keep in mind that they require soaking overnight. You can skip this step, but you won't get the rich vanilla flavor if you do. It's better to prepare in advance and start soaking the day before you want to make the nuts.*

**Serves 6**

1 tablespoon pure vanilla extract
½ cup water
½ cup crushed raw cashews
½ cup crushed raw almonds
1 tablespoon ground cinnamon
1 teaspoon ground nutmeg

**1** Combine vanilla extract and water in a medium mixing bowl and stir. Add nuts and allow to soak 12 hours or overnight. Remove nuts from water and spread out on a paper towel. Allow to dry 3 hours.

**2** Preheat oven to 200°F. Line baking sheet with parchment paper.

**3** Place nuts in a medium bowl and add cinnamon and nutmeg. Toss to coat.

**4** Spread nuts out on lined baking sheet and bake 3 hours. Remove from oven and allow to cool.

**5** Transfer to an airtight container and store until ready to eat.

**Per Serving**
Calories: 131 | Fat: 9.3 g | Protein: 4.2 g | Sodium: 1 mg | Fiber: 2.3 g | Carbohydrates: 7.2 g | Net Carbohydrates: 4.9 g | Sugar: 1.4 g

# MAPLE NUT BARS

*This recipe calls for stevia-sweetened maple syrup, not sugar-free maple syrup. Try to avoid the latter, which is typically sweetened with artificial sweeteners that have been linked to negative health effects.*

**Serves 6**

1 cup raw almonds
½ cup raw cashews
¾ cup raw macadamia nuts
½ cup no-sugar-added creamy almond butter
⅓ cup stevia-sweetened maple syrup
⅛ teaspoon salt

**1** Add nuts to the bowl of a food processor and pulse until a crumbly mixture forms (but not so much that they turn into flour).

**2** Transfer to a medium mixing bowl and combine nuts with almond butter, maple syrup, and salt.

**3** Line an 8" × 8" baking pan with parchment paper and press mixture into pan. Place in the refrigerator and allow to set 2 hours or until bars are hardened.

**4** Cut into 6 equal portions and store in the refrigerator until ready to eat.

**Per Serving**
Calories: 498 | Fat: 39.3 g | Protein: 12.6 g | Sodium: 52 mg | Fiber: 6.8 g | Carbohydrates: 28.2 g | Net Carbohydrates: 21.4 g | Sugar: 13.1 g

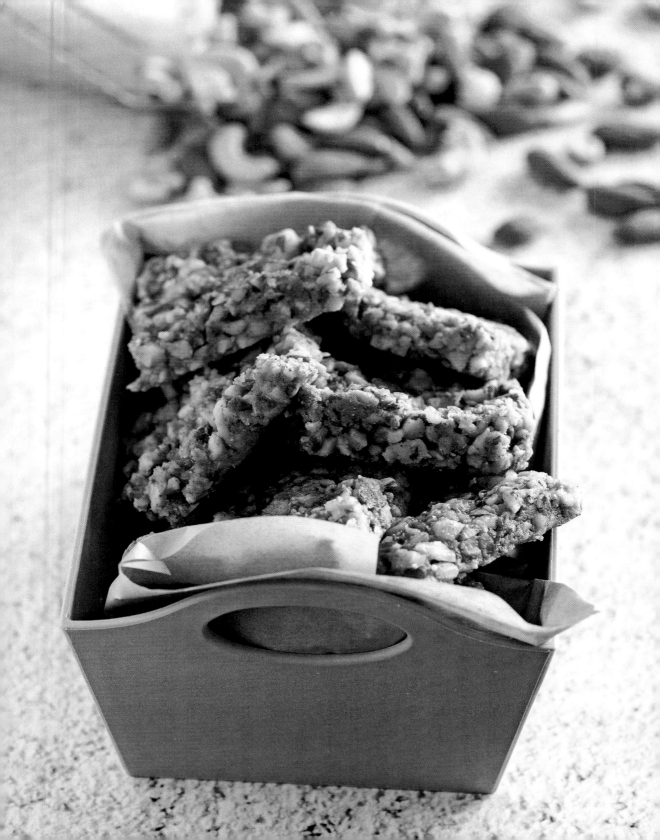

# CACAO TRAIL MIX

*If you want to kick the flavor of this trail mix up a notch, you can toast the coconut flakes before mixing them in with the nuts. Just arrange them on a baking sheet and bake at 325°F for 10 minutes and then follow the rest of the recipe as written.*

**Serves 6**

½ cup chopped walnuts
½ cup shelled pistachios
½ cup sprouted pumpkin seeds
¼ cup cashew pieces
½ cup cacao nibs
½ cup unsweetened coconut flakes

**1** Combine all ingredients in a medium bowl and toss to combine.

**2** Store in an airtight container until ready to eat.

**Per Serving**
Calories: 341 | Fat: 27.5 g | Protein: 9.1 g | Sodium: 14 mg | Fiber: 7.0 g | Carbohydrates: 16.0 g | Net Carbohydrates: 9.0 g | Sugar: 3.2 g

## Cacao versus Cocoa

Raw cacao powder is made by cold-pressing unroasted cocoa beans, which keeps the beneficial enzymes intact. Cocoa powder is raw cacao powder that has been roasted at low temperatures. This roasting process makes cocoa sweeter tasting but destroys some of the antioxidants and nutrients.

# COCONUT CHIA SMOOTHIE

*You can turn this into a chocolate coconut chia smoothie by adding a couple of tablespoons of unsweetened cocoa powder before blending.*

**Serves 1**

**1 cup full-fat canned coconut milk**
**2 tablespoons chia seeds**
**2 tablespoons coconut oil, melted**
**¼ cup frozen blueberries**

**1** Place all ingredients in a blender and blend until smooth.

**2** Serve cold.

**Per Serving**
Calories: 843 | Fat: 79.8 g | Protein: 10.0 g | Sodium: 33 mg | Fiber: 11.4 g | Carbohydrates: 23.7 g | Net Carbohydrates: 12.3 g | Sugar: 3.3 g

## Choosing Coconut Milk

The coconut milk that comes in a box is full of preservatives and low in fat. Some sweetened varieties contain sugar or other sweeteners that increase carbohydrate content. Look for full-fat coconut milk in a can that contains only coconut milk or a combination of coconut milk and guar gum.

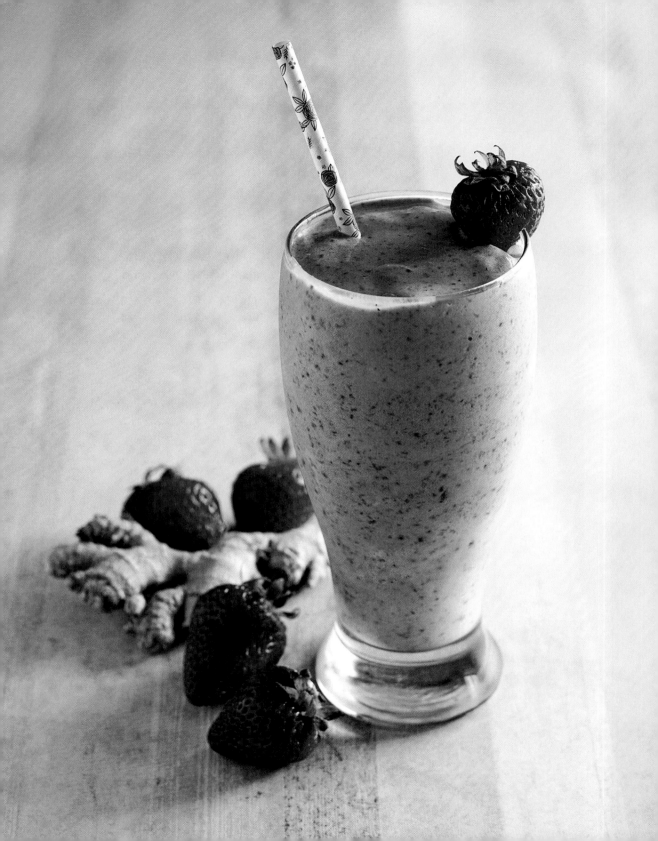

# GINGER STRAWBERRY SMOOTHIE

*The soothing effects of ginger make this recipe perfect for optimizing digestion. If you prefer a thicker, colder shake, add crushed ice ½ cup at a time until suitably thick and creamy.*

**Serves 4**

1 cup watercress
¾ cup frozen strawberries
½" piece gingerroot, peeled
1 cup full-fat canned coconut milk
1 cup heavy cream, divided

**1** Combine watercress, strawberries, ginger, coconut milk, and ½ cup heavy cream in a blender and blend until thoroughly combined.

**2** Add remaining heavy cream as needed while blending until desired consistency is reached.

**Per Serving**
Calories: 327 | Fat: 32.2 g | Protein: 2.7 g | Sodium: 33 mg | Fiber: 0.6 g | Carbohydrates: 6.0 g | Net Carbohydrates: 5.4 g | Sugar: 3.0 g

# COCOA COCONUT BUTTER FAT BOMBS

*In addition to coconut oil, this recipe uses coconut butter, which differs from the oil. Coconut butter is the puréed meat of mature coconuts, while coconut oil has been separated from the coconut meat. One cannot be substituted for the other.*

**Serves 12**

1 cup coconut oil
½ cup unsalted butter
6 tablespoons unsweetened cocoa powder
15 drops liquid stevia
½ cup coconut butter

**Make Your Own**

Coconut butter isn't always easy to find. It's simple and more cost-effective to make your own. To make 2 cups of coconut butter, put 6 cups of unsweetened coconut flakes into a blender with a pinch of salt and blend until completely smooth. This usually takes 5–6 minutes.

**1** Put coconut oil, butter, cocoa powder, and stevia in a small saucepan over low heat, stirring frequently until all ingredients are melted.

**2** Melt coconut butter in a separate small pan over low heat.

**3** Pour 2 tablespoons of cocoa mixture into each well of a 12-cup silicone mold.

**4** Add 1 tablespoon of melted coconut butter to each well.

**5** Place in the freezer until hardened, about 30 minutes.

**6** Store in the refrigerator until ready to eat.

**Per Serving**
Calories: 297 | Fat: 30.6 g | Protein: 1.3 g | Sodium: 4 mg | Fiber: 2.3 g | Carbohydrates: 3.6 g | Net Carbohydrates: 1.3 g | Sugar: 0.7 g

# COFFEE COCONUT BERRY SMOOTHIE

*For a different flavor, use blueberries or blackberries in place of the raspberries (or a combination of all three).*

**Serves 2**

1 cup full-fat canned coconut milk
1 cup brewed coffee
2 tablespoons unsweetened cocoa powder
¼ cup frozen raspberries
1 tablespoon granulated erythritol
2 tablespoons no-sugar-added cashew butter

Put all ingredients in a blender and blend until smooth.

**Per Serving**
Calories: 338 | Fat: 30.9 g | Protein: 6.5 g | Sodium: 19 mg | Fiber: 3.5 g | Carbohydrates: 20.3 g | Net Carbohydrates: 9.3 g | Sugar Alcohols: 7.5 g | Sugar: 0.9 g

# RASPBERRY CHEESECAKE FAT BOMBS

*You can replace the raspberries in this recipe with blackberries, blueberries, or strawberries. Combine them all for a delicious mixed-berry cheesecake bomb.*

**Serves 12**

½ cup frozen raspberries

10 drops liquid stevia

1 teaspoon vanilla extract

6 ounces (¾ cup) cream cheese, softened to room temperature

¼ cup coconut oil, softened

**1** Place raspberries in a food processer and process until smooth. Add stevia and vanilla extract and process until incorporated.

**2** Add cream cheese and coconut oil and process until all ingredients are well combined.

**3** Place an equal amount of mixture in each well of a 12-cup silicone mold.

**4** Place in freezer until hardened, about 30 minutes.

**5** Store in the refrigerator until ready to eat.

**Per Serving**
Calories: 91 | Fat: 8.4 g | Protein: 0.9 g | Sodium: 51 mg | Fiber: 0.4 g | Carbohydrates: 1.3 g | Net Carbohydrates: 0.9 g | Sugar: 0.8 g

## Be Careful with Berries

Berries are full of fiber, so their net carbohydrate count is not as high as some other fruits. In fact, 1 cup contains 7 net carbohydrates. You still need to be careful when eating berries on a ketogenic diet. Don't overdo it and always make sure to count your macronutrients to make sure that berries fit into your plan that day.

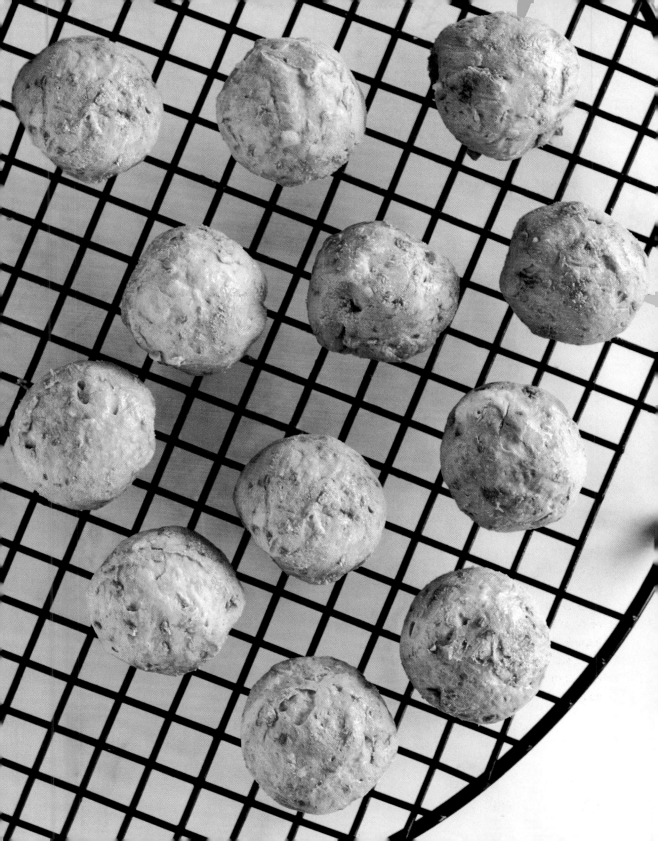

# DARK CHOCOLATE ESPRESSO FAT BOMBS

*Who doesn't love the flavors of chocolate and coffee together? These fat bombs will give you energy without all the caffeine!*

**Makes 8 fat bombs**

2 tablespoons cocoa butter

2 tablespoons coconut oil

2 ounces dark unsweetened baking chocolate

¼ teaspoon coffee extract

5 drops stevia glycerite

**1** In a small saucepan over very low heat, add cocoa butter, coconut oil, and chocolate, stirring until completely melted, about 3 minutes.

**2** Remove from heat and stir in coffee extract and stevia.

**3** Pour into 8 silicone molds. Refrigerate until hard.

**4** Remove from molds. Serve immediately or store in refrigerator up to 1 week.

**Per Serving**
Calories: 104 | Fat: 10.0 g | Protein: 1.0 g | Sodium: 1 mg | Fiber: 1.2 g | Carbohydrates: 2.0 g | Net Carbohydrates: 0.8 g | Sugar: 0.0 g

# MIXED-NUT GRAIN-FREE GRANOLA BARS

*These treats are as tasty as granola bars without any of the grains or sugar. Another excellent addition to consider would be freeze-dried raspberries or blueberries.*

**Makes 14 fat bombs**

½ cup pumpkin seeds
½ cup sunflower seeds
½ cup coarsely chopped almonds
¼ cup unsweetened shredded coconut
¼ cup coconut oil, melted
4 tablespoons no-sugar-added almond butter
1 teaspoon vanilla extract
2 teaspoons ground cinnamon
⅛ teaspoon salt
3 tablespoons granular Swerve sweetener
2 large eggs

**1** Preheat oven to 350°F.

**2** Place seeds and almonds in food processor and pulse to break them up slightly.

**3** Add remaining ingredients and pulse until well combined.

**4** Spread mixture into an 8" × 8" silicone baking dish (or a glass dish lightly greased with coconut oil).

**5** Bake 20 minutes.

**6** Allow to cool and cut into 14 equal bars before serving.

**Per Serving**
Calories: 165 | Fat: 14.4 g | Protein: 5.0 g | Sodium: 31 mg | Fiber: 2.3 g | Carbohydrates: 7.8 g | Net Carbohydrates: 2.3 g | Sugar Alcohols: 3.2 g | Sugar: 0.5 g

## The Great Granola Debate

While many health-food lovers believe granola to be an excellent nutrient-packed snack, others in the nutrition industry believe otherwise. Traditional granola bars, though full of fiber and iron from the granola as well as healthy fats from the seeds and nuts, are also filled with alarming amounts of sugar, making them a less-than-healthy choice.

# SALTED CARAMEL AND PECAN TRUFFLES

*These truffles are quite indulgent. Keep them for those moments when you feel you need a special treat.*

**Makes 9 fat bombs**

2 ounces unsweetened baking chocolate

1 tablespoon butter

1 tablespoon cream cheese

2 tablespoons confectioners' Swerve

2 drops stevia glycerite

½ teaspoon liquid caramel flavor

½ teaspoon sea salt

3 tablespoons chopped pecans

**1** In a small double boiler over medium-low heat, melt chocolate while slowly stirring.

**2** Add butter, cream cheese, Swerve, stevia, caramel flavor, and salt to chocolate and mix well until incorporated.

**3** Remove from heat and keep stirring about 10 seconds.

**4** Place saucepan in refrigerator about 1 hour until ganache has solidified.

**5** Scoop ganache with a spoon and form 9 little balls. You might want to wear plastic gloves to help keep the chocolate from sticking to your hands.

**6** Place chopped pecans on a medium plate and roll truffles through to coat evenly.

**Per Serving**
Calories: 72 | Fat: 6.4 g | Protein: 1.2 g | Sodium: 94 mg | Fiber: 1.3 g | Carbohydrates: 4.2 g | Net Carbohydrates: 0.9 g | Sugar Alcohols: 2.0 g | Sugar: 0.2 g

# COCONUT VANILLA POPSICLES

*A simple, clean flavor to please even the pickiest eaters. Kids will love these popsicles.*

**Makes 8 fat bombs**

2 cups unsweetened coconut cream, chilled
¼ cup unsweetened shredded coconut
1 teaspoon vanilla extract
¼ cup erythritol or granular Swerve

**1** Place all ingredients in a blender and blend until completely mixed, about 30 seconds.

**2** Pour mix into 8 popsicle molds, tapping molds to dislodge air bubbles.

**3** Freeze at least 8 hours or overnight.

**4** Remove popsicles from molds. If popsicles are hard to remove, run molds under hot water briefly, and popsicles will come loose.

**Per Serving**
Calories: 214 | Fat: 21.1 g | Protein: 2.3 g | Sodium: 2 mg | Fiber: 1.8 g | Carbohydrates: 12.2 g | Net Carbohydrates: 2.9 g | Sugar Alcohols: 7.5 g | Sugar: 0.2 g

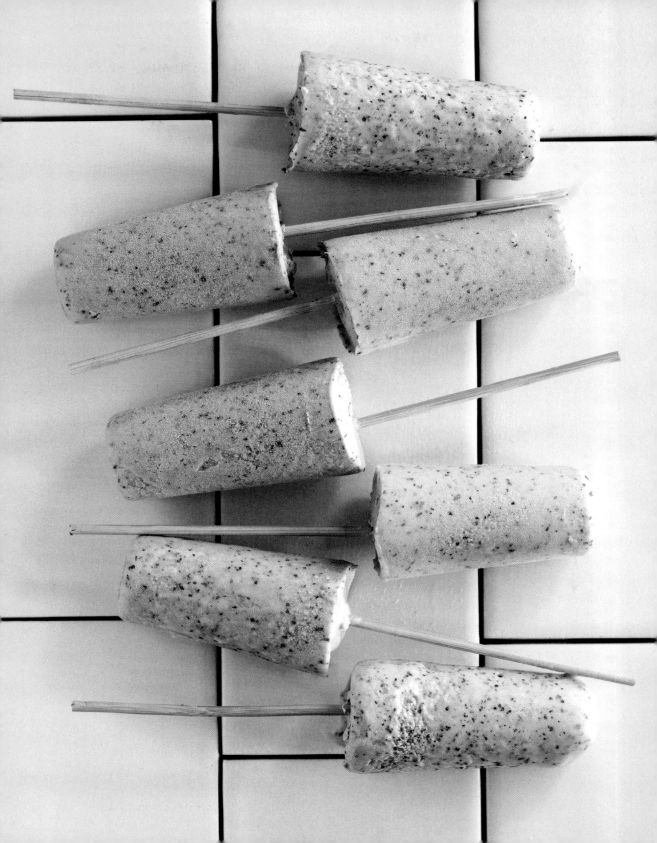

# MATCHA POPSICLES

*Creamy, refreshing, and with the energizing qualities of matcha, these are delicious popsicles for grownups.*

**Makes 8 fat bombs**

**2 cups unsweetened coconut cream, chilled**
**2 tablespoons coconut oil**
**1 teaspoon matcha**
**¼ cup erythritol or granular Swerve**

**1** Place all ingredients in a blender and blend until completely mixed, about 30 seconds.

**2** Pour mix into 8 popsicle molds, tapping molds to dislodge air bubbles.

**3** Freeze at least 8 hours or overnight.

**4** Remove popsicles from molds. If popsicles are hard to remove, run molds under hot water briefly, and popsicles will come loose.

## Green Rocket Fuel

Matcha is a finely ground powder of a specially grown green tea. Matcha is basically a form of whole green tea leaves with extra theanine and chlorophyll. It also contains high levels of catechin antioxidants and a good amount of caffeine. As matcha contains the whole leaf, you also get a higher content of nutrients than in regular brewed green tea.

**Per Serving**
Calories: 227 | Fat: 22.8 g | Protein: 2.2 g | Sodium: 2 mg | Fiber: 1.4 g | Carbohydrates: 11.6 g | Net Carbohydrates: 2.7 g | Sugar Alcohols: 7.5 g | Sugar: 0.0 g

# CINNAMON BUN FAT BOMBS

*These Cinnamon Bun Fat Bombs have the same flavor as a cinnamon roll fresh from the oven but without the sugar and carbohydrates.*

**Serves 12**

1 cup coconut butter, softened

¼ teaspoon plus ⅛ teaspoon ground cinnamon, divided

¼ teaspoon ground nutmeg

¼ teaspoon vanilla extract

¼ cup crushed walnuts

**1** Combine coconut butter, ¼ teaspoon cinnamon, nutmeg, and vanilla extract in a small bowl and mix until well combined.

**2** Separate the mixture into 12 equal parts and roll into balls. Place on a cookie sheet lined with wax paper.

**3** Mix crushed walnuts with remaining cinnamon in a small bowl. Roll balls in nut mixture until coated.

**4** Place finished balls on a cookie sheet lined with wax paper and refrigerate until ready to eat.

## Smooth It Out

The crushed walnuts finish off these fat bombs with a nice crunch, but you could also grind the walnuts instead for a smooth but still decadent finish.

**Per Serving**
Calories: 149 | Fat: 13.5 g | Protein: 1.7 g | Sodium: 6 mg | Fiber: 2.9 g | Carbohydrates: 4.4 g | Net Carbohydrates: 1.5 g | Sugar: 1.4 g

# TOASTED COCONUT BARK

*Although delicious with regular shredded coconut, toasting the shaved coconut meat adds an extra nutty flavor that's hard to beat. The addition of another tropical nut elevates this bark to divine.*

**Serves 12**

⅓ cup unsweetened coconut flakes
1 cup coconut oil
¼ cup confectioners' Swerve
⅔ cup coarsely chopped macadamia nuts

**1** Line an 8" × 8" pan with parchment paper.

**2** In a small nonstick pan over medium heat, toast coconut flakes just until meat turns light brown, about 5 minutes. Set aside.

**3** Combine coconut oil and Swerve in a small saucepan over medium heat, stirring frequently until melted. Turn off heat.

**4** Add coconut flakes and nuts to saucepan and stir.

**5** Pour mixture into lined pan and spread it out with the back of a wooden spoon.

**6** Freeze or refrigerate to set bark.

**7** Break bark into chunks before serving.

## Macadamia Madness

Macadamia nuts have grown so much in popularity that California decided to get in on the growing action in the late 1980s. While the trees take 4–5 years to produce nuts, they were an excellent investment for the warm climate in the southwestern states. Hawaii, however, is still the largest producer of these tasty nuts.

**Per Serving**
Calories: 224 | Fat: 23.8 g | Protein: 0.7 g | Sodium: 0 mg | Fiber: 1.1 g | Carbohydrates: 4.6 g | Net Carbohydrates: 0.3 g | Sugar Alcohols: 3.0 g | Sugar: 0.5 g

# CHOCOLATE ORANGE FAT BOMBS

*The citrus notes in the orange extract in this recipe bring out the flavor of the unsweetened cocoa powder. You can make this a double-chocolate fat bomb instead by swapping out the orange extract for chocolate extract.*

**Serves 12**

½ cup unsalted butter
½ cup coconut oil
5 tablespoons unsweetened cocoa powder
1 teaspoon orange extract

**1** Mix all ingredients together in a small saucepan over medium-low heat until melted and smooth.

**2** Pour into a 12-cup silicone mold and place into the freezer until hardened, about 30 minutes.

**3** Store in the refrigerator until ready to eat.

**Per Serving**
Calories: 152 | Fat: 16.0 g | Protein: 0.5 g | Sodium: 1 mg | Fiber: 0.8 g | Carbohydrates: 1.4 g | Net Carbohydrates: 0.6 g | Sugar: 0.1 g

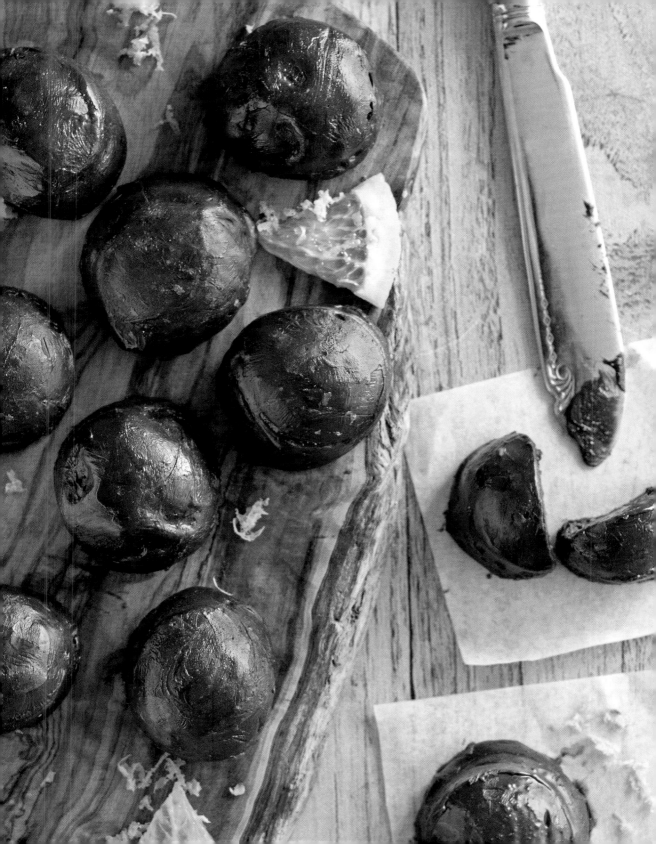

# EGGNOG FUDGE

*Nothing says holidays like the creamy, old-fashioned flavor of eggnog. While an excellent fat bomb on its own, eggnog is usually too full of sugar to make it a worthwhile treat for a low-carb, high-fat dieter. Now you can enjoy the flavor of the holidays without the sugar overload.*

**Makes 4 fat bombs**

8 tablespoons butter
4 ounces (½ cup) cream cheese, softened
1 tablespoon vanilla extract
1 teaspoon ground nutmeg
¼ teaspoon ground cinnamon
⅛ teaspoon ground cloves
2 tablespoons granular Swerve

**1** Grease and line a 9" × 5" loaf pan with parchment paper.

**2** In a medium saucepan over medium-low heat, melt butter. Add cream cheese and stir until melted and combined.

**3** Remove from heat, add remaining ingredients, and mix well.

**4** Spread mixture into lined loaf pan.

**5** Let cool to room temperature, then place in refrigerator to finish setting, at least 2 hours.

**6** Slice into 4 pieces before serving.

**Per Serving**
Calories: 312 | Fat: 29.9 g | Protein: 2.0 g | Sodium: 106 mg | Fiber: 0.2 g | Carbohydrates: 9.5 g | Net Carbohydrates: 1.8 g | Sugar Alcohols: 7.5 g | Sugar: 1.4 g

## How Did Eggnog Get Its Name?

While the origin of the drink is still up for debate, the name *eggnog* most likely comes from the small wooden cup it was originally served in, known as a noggin.

# CHOCOLATE CARAMEL FAT BOMBS

*These are creamy, chocolaty fat bombs with the flavor of caramel. The flavor is pretty darn close to candy!*

**Makes 12 fat bombs**

6 tablespoons coconut oil

6 tablespoons heavy cream

2 ounces dark unsweetened baking chocolate

2 tablespoons caramel extract

2 tablespoons confectioners' Swerve

**1** In a small saucepan over very low heat, add all the ingredients, stirring until completely melted. Pour into 12 silicone molds.

**2** Refrigerate until hard. Remove from molds. Serve immediately or store in refrigerator up to 1 week.

**Per Serving**
Calories: 114 | Fat: 11.4 g | Protein: 0.8 g | Sodium: 3 mg | Fiber: 0.8 g | Carbohydrates: 3.6 g | Net Carbohydrates: 0.3 g | Sugar Alcohols: 2.5 g | Sugar: 0.3 g

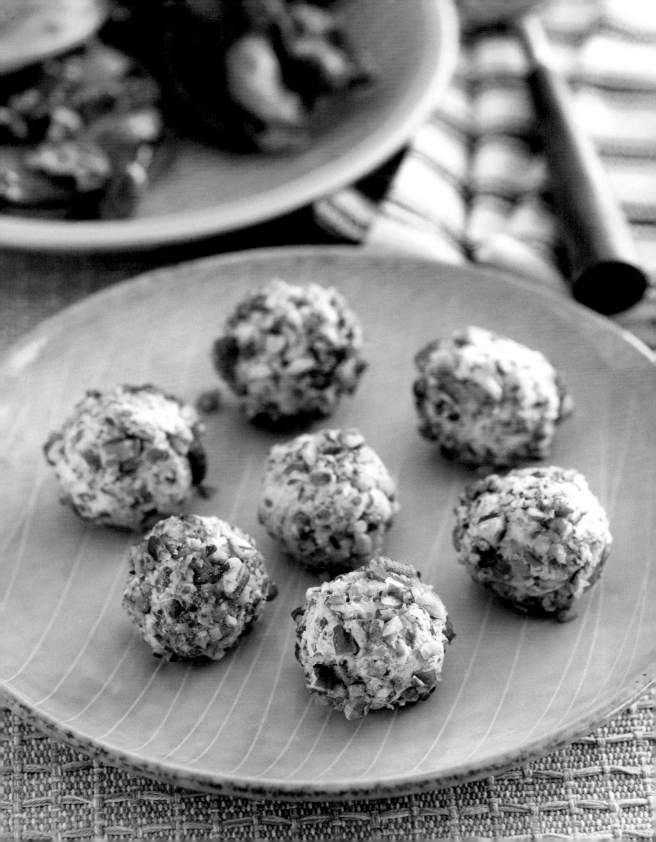

# BACON MAPLE PANCAKE BALLS

*These fat bombs have the flavor of breakfast pancakes with maple syrup and bacon. They're a great way to start the day off right!*

**Makes 6 fat bombs**

**5 slices no-sugar-added bacon, cooked**
**4 ounces (½ cup) cream cheese**
**½ teaspoon maple flavor**
**¼ teaspoon salt**
**3 tablespoons crushed pecans**

**1** On a cutting board, chop bacon into small crumbs.

**2** In a small bowl, combine cream cheese and bacon crumbles with maple flavor and salt; mix well with a fork.

**3** Form mixture into 6 balls.

**4** Place crushed pecans on a medium plate and roll individual balls through to coat evenly.

**5** Serve immediately or refrigerate up to 3 days.

## Food Flavoring versus Sugar-Free Syrup

A lot of recipes on the ketogenic diet call for sugar-free syrup. Such syrups contain ingredients like acesulfame potassium, sodium hexametaphosphate, and phosphoric acid. Those artificial flavors, preservatives, and fillers are not health-building ingredients; on the contrary, they load the body with toxins. A good organic maple flavor will only contain a maple distillate and pure grain alcohol.

**Per Serving**
Calories: 132 | Fat: 11.1 g | Protein: 4.7 g | Sodium: 327 mg | Fiber: 0.3 g | Carbohydrates: 1.4 g | Net Carbohydrates: 1.1 g | Sugar: 0.7 g

# CHOCOLATE MOUSSE

*You'll love this mousse so much you won't even miss the real thing. The avocado adds healthy fats, but the taste is camouflaged by the cocoa powder.*

**Serves 4**

4 ounces (½ cup) cream cheese, softened
½ cup unsalted butter, softened
2 tablespoons granulated erythritol
½ large avocado, peeled and pitted
2 tablespoons unsweetened cocoa powder
⅔ cup heavy cream

**1** Beat cream cheese, butter, and granulated erythritol together in a medium bowl until light and fluffy.

**2** Add avocado and cocoa powder and beat until smooth. Stir in heavy cream.

**3** Divide into 4 serving dishes and refrigerate until chilled, about 30 minutes. Serve cold.

**Per Serving**
Calories: 471 | Fat: 46.3 g | Protein: 3.6 g | Sodium: 123 mg | Fiber: 2.2 g | Carbohydrates: 12.8 g | Net Carbohydrates: 3.1 g | Sugar Alcohols: 7.5 g | Sugar: 2.1 g

## Whip Up Some Cream

You can turn this from a snack into dessert by whipping up some coconut cream to put on top. Simply take the coconut cream from a can of coconut milk that's been refrigerated for 24 hours, add a couple of tablespoons of powdered erythritol and a teaspoon of vanilla extract, and beat for 2–4 minutes or until cream is light and fluffy.

# KALE AND BRAZIL NUT SMOOTHIE

*This unusual blend of ingredients delivers sound nutrition and unique flavor. Kale is a nutritional powerhouse that provides an abundance of vitamins A and K. Ninety-one percent of Brazil nuts' calories come from fat, making them a perfect addition to the ketogenic diet.*

**Serves 2**

2 cups chopped kale
¼ cup Brazil nuts, frozen
2 tablespoons coconut oil, melted
2 cups full-fat canned coconut milk
½ teaspoon ground cinnamon
½ teaspoon ground allspice
½–1 cup ice, as needed

**1** Place kale, nuts, coconut oil, coconut milk, cinnamon, and allspice in a blender and blend until thoroughly combined.

**2** With the blender running, add ice in small batches until desired consistency is reached. If smoothie is too thick, add splashes of water to thin out the consistency.

**Per Serving**
Calories: 681 | Fat: 68.9 g | Protein: 7.7 g | Sodium: 35 mg | Fiber: 2.3 g | Carbohydrates: 10.6 g | Net Carbohydrates: 8.3 g | Sugar: 0.8 g

## Brazil Nut Ecology

Brazil nuts grow on large, old-growth trees in the Amazon. These trees can live to be 500 years old. Brazil nuts are one of the Amazon's potentially sustainable resources because they can be harvested each year without damaging the trees, but the nut production requires a delicate environmental balance that is being threatened by deforestation.

# PUMPKIN FAT BOMBS

*For a richer taste, swap out the coconut oil in this recipe for unsalted butter. Keep the amount of coconut butter the same.*

**Serves 12**

½ cup coconut butter, softened
¼ cup coconut oil, softened
⅛ cup pumpkin purée
1 teaspoon pumpkin pie spice
¼ teaspoon vanilla extract
8 drops liquid stevia
⅛ teaspoon salt

**1** Mix all ingredients together in a small bowl and stir until combined.

**2** Pour into an 8" × 8" baking pan and spread mixture out evenly. Refrigerate 30 minutes and then cut into 12 squares.

**Per Serving**
Calories: 106 | Fat: 10.3 g | Protein: 0.7 g | Sodium: 27 mg | Fiber: 1.4 g | Carbohydrates: 2.2 g | Net Carbohydrates: 0.8 g | Sugar: 0.8 g

### Go for the Gourd

Canned pumpkin is about 90 percent water, so it contains very few calories—fewer than 50 per serving. Pumpkin is also rich in fiber, containing 7 grams per cup, but it's not considered a low-carbohydrate food. Pumpkin can be incorporated into a ketogenic diet, but always watch your portions.

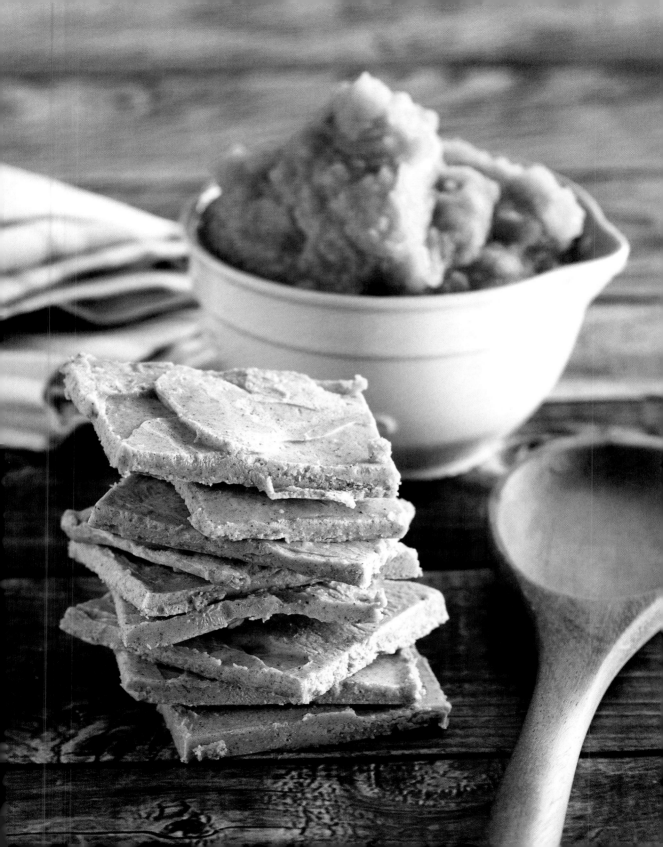

# CALMING CUCUMBER SMOOTHIE

*The light taste of cucumber and the refreshing fragrance of mint combine with romaine lettuce in this delightful smoothie. Toasted almonds make a great addition to this smoothie; try adding a tablespoon of sliced toasted almonds in addition to the coconut flakes.*

**Serves 4**

1 cup chopped romaine lettuce
2 medium cucumbers, peeled
¼ cup chopped mint
1 cup full-fat canned coconut milk, divided
¼ cup unsweetened coconut flakes

**1** Combine romaine, cucumbers, mint, and ½ cup coconut milk in a blender and combine thoroughly.

**2** Add remaining coconut milk while blending.

**3** Divide smoothie mixture into 4 glasses. Top each glass with 1 tablespoon coconut flakes to garnish.

**Per Serving**
Calories: 159 | Fat: 14.4 g | Protein: 2.3 g | Sodium: 10 mg | Fiber: 2.1 g | Carbohydrates: 5.7 g | Net Carbohydrates: 3.6 g | Sugar: 1.9 g

## Cucumbers Aren't Just Water

Even though a cucumber is mostly water (and fiber), it is far more than a tasty, thirst-quenching, and filling snack option. These green veggies have detoxifying and rehydrating properties. By consuming one serving of cucumber per day, you'll not only fulfill a full serving of veggies and stave off hunger; you'll have clear, hydrated skin!

# AVOCADO FAT BOMB SMOOTHIE

*The avocado in this recipe will make your smoothie nice and creamy without changing the flavor.*

**Serves 2**

1 cup full-fat canned coconut milk
½ large avocado, peeled and pitted
¼ cup ice
1 teaspoon vanilla extract
1 tablespoon granulated erythritol
2 tablespoons coconut butter

Combine all ingredients in blender and blend until smooth. Serve immediately.

**Per Serving**
Calories: 385 | Fat: 36.3 g | Protein: 4.0 g | Sodium: 22 mg | Fiber: 4.3 g | Carbohydrates: 16.9 g | Net Carbohydrates: 5.1 g | Sugar Alcohols: 7.5 g | Sugar: 1.4 g

# SUNBUTTER BALLS

*This recipe could also be called the Cravings Killer, as it can help curb your sugar cravings naturally!*

**Makes 12 fat bombs**

**6 tablespoons mascarpone cheese**

**3 tablespoons no-sugar-added sunflower seed butter**

**6 tablespoons coconut oil, softened**

**3 tablespoons unsweetened shredded coconut flakes**

**1** In a medium bowl, mix mascarpone cheese, sunflower seed butter, and coconut oil until a smooth paste forms.

**2** Shape paste into walnut-sized balls. If mixture is too sticky, place in refrigerator 15 minutes before forming balls.

**3** Spread coconut flakes on a medium plate and roll individual balls through to coat evenly.

**Per Serving**
Calories: 114 | Fat: 8.1 g | Protein: 1.5 g | Sodium: 16 mg | Fiber: 0.5 g | Carbohydrates: 1.5 g | Net Carbohydrates: 1.0 g | Sugar: 0.5 g

## An Italian Delight

Mascarpone is an Italian soft cheese best known for being used in the famous tiramisu. It is actually the perfect ingredient for fat bombs; it's creamy, delicious, and contains zero carbs!

# ALMOND BUTTER MUFFINS

*For some variety, replace the almond butter in this recipe with another one of your favorite nut butters. Cashew butter, peanut butter, and sunflower seed butter work well.*

**Serves 12**

⅔ cup almond flour
¼ cup granulated erythritol
1 teaspoon ground cinnamon
¼ cup no-sugar-added almond butter
2 tablespoons butter
1 tablespoon coconut oil
1 teaspoon vanilla extract
4 large eggs
¼ cup heavy cream

**1** Preheat oven to 350°F.

**2** Mix together almond flour, erythritol, and cinnamon in a medium mixing bowl.

**3** In a separate large bowl, beat almond butter, butter, coconut oil, vanilla extract, eggs, and cream together until smooth.

**4** Add almond flour mixture to almond butter mixture and stir until smooth.

**5** Put a paper cupcake liner in each well of a 12-cup muffin tin. Fill each paper cup with batter.

**6** Bake 20 minutes or until a toothpick inserted in the center comes out clean.

**7** Remove cups from muffin tin and allow to cool before serving.

## Learning about Erythritol

Erythritol is a naturally derived sugar substitute that looks and tastes like sugar but has almost no calories and a low glycemic load, which means it doesn't significantly affect your blood sugar levels. Erythritol comes in two forms, granulated and powdered, and can be used in place of sugar in any recipe.

**Per Serving**
Calories: 136 | Fat: 11.9 g | Protein: 4.6 g | Sodium: 25 mg | Fiber: 1.3 g | Carbohydrates: 8.2 g | Net Carbohydrates: 2.2 g | Sugar Alcohols: 5.0 g | Sugar: 0.5 g

# PEANUT BUTTER CREAM CHEESE FAT BOMBS

*The crunchy peanut butter and crushed peanuts in this recipe give these fat bombs an unbeatable texture. If you prefer less crunch, use smooth peanut butter instead.*

**Makes 12 fat bombs**

1 cup coconut oil

½ cup butter

½ cup no-sugar-added crunchy peanut butter

2 tablespoons cream cheese

10 drops liquid stevia

¼ cup crushed unsalted peanuts

**1** Place coconut oil, butter, peanut butter, cream cheese, and stevia in a small saucepan over medium heat and stir until melted.

**2** Sprinkle crushed peanuts evenly in each well of a 12-cup mini muffin pan lined with cupcake wrappers. Pour peanut butter mixture over peanuts.

**3** Place in freezer until hardened, about 30 minutes.

**4** Store in refrigerator up to 1 week.

**Per Serving**
Calories: 313 | Fat: 31.6 g | Protein: 3.6 g | Sodium: 9 mg | Fiber: 1.3 g | Carbohydrates: 3.1 g | Net Carbohydrates: 1.8 g | Sugar: 0.6 g

# CINNAMON ROLL BARS

*With all the flavor of a cinnamon roll and none of the gluten or sugar, these treats are sure to please even the strongest sweet tooth.*

**Makes 4 fat bombs**

1 cup creamed coconut, cut into chunks
1¼ teaspoons ground cinnamon, divided
2 tablespoons coconut oil
2 tablespoons no-sugar-added almond butter

**1** Line a mini loaf pan with parchment paper or loaf pan liners.

**2** In a medium bowl, mix creamed coconut and ¼ teaspoon cinnamon with hands thoroughly and press into bottom of loaf pan.

**3** In a small bowl, whisk coconut oil, almond butter, and 1 teaspoon cinnamon until combined and then spread over creamed coconut layer.

**4** Place pan in freezer 10 minutes to set.

**5** Cut into 4 equal-sized fat bombs and eat immediately.

## Health Benefits of Cinnamon

Filled with antioxidants and anti-inflammatory in nature, cinnamon makes an excellent addition to any diet. Cinnamon is known to curb hunger, lower blood pressure, and reduce the risk of heart disease.

**Per Serving**
Calories: 268 | Fat: 26.5 g | Protein: 3.1 g | Sodium: 8 mg | Fiber: 4.4 g | Carbohydrates: 9.1 g | Net Carbohydrates: 4.7 g | Sugar: 1.6 g

# WHITE CHOCOLATE PECAN FAT BOMBS

*This classic fat-bomb recipe is easy and incredibly delicious. Walnuts would be a great addition if you're out of pecans.*

**Makes 8 fat bombs**

¼ cup pecans
4 tablespoons cocoa butter
4 tablespoons coconut oil
¼ teaspoon vanilla extract
5 drops stevia glycerite

**1** Chop pecans coarsely with a knife or process quickly in a food processor so they don't get too fine.

**2** In a small saucepan over very low heat, add cocoa butter and coconut oil, stirring until completely melted, about 3 minutes.

**3** Remove from heat and stir in pecans, vanilla extract, and stevia.

**4** Pour into 8 silicone molds. Refrigerate until hard.

**5** Remove from molds. Serve immediately or store in refrigerator up to 1 week.

## Be Choosy with Nuts

When buying nuts, opt for raw, unsalted varieties rather than roasted, salted, or sugared versions. Raw nuts generally contain no added ingredients while roasted, flavored nuts can contain unhealthy oils and sugar.

**Per Serving**
Calories: 142 | Fat: 15.3 g | Protein: 0.3 g | Sodium: 0 mg | Fiber: 0.3 g | Carbohydrates: 0.5 g | Net Carbohydrates: 0.2 g | Sugar: 0.2 g

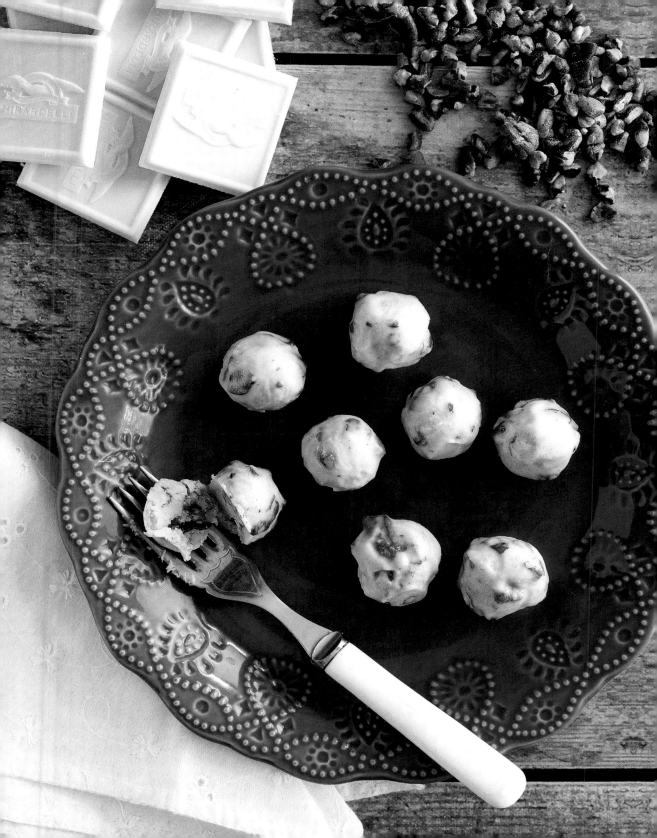

# TURMERIC-INFUSED PANNA COTTA

*Turmeric used to be considered an exotic spice, but it is now widely available in any supermarket, even the fresh root version. Try this pungent condiment, and the earthy but distinct flavor will surely win you over.*

**Makes 6 fat bombs**

**1½ cups full-fat canned coconut milk, refrigerated and cream separated from the water**

**1½ cups beef stock**

**1½ tablespoons powdered unflavored gelatin**

**1 tablespoon turmeric**

**½ tablespoon sea salt**

**1** In a small saucepan over medium heat, heat coconut cream and beef stock.

**2** Whisk in gelatin until completely incorporated.

**3** Add turmeric and salt and simmer 5 minutes.

**4** Pour mixture evenly into 6 small glasses or ramekins. Refrigerate until set, at least 6 hours or overnight.

**5** Serve in glass or ramekin or invert over a small plate after dipping glass or ramekin into hot water a few seconds.

## The Benefits of Turmeric

The main active ingredient in turmeric, called curcumin (not to be confused with the common spice cumin), is recognized as being a powerful anti-inflammatory. Even a small serving in a dish can assist your body's ability to digest fats and reduce bloating.

**Per Serving**
Calories: 129 | Fat: 11.4 g | Protein: 4.0 g | Sodium: 259 mg | Fiber: 0.4 g | Carbohydrates: 3.4 g | Net Carbohydrates: 3.0 g | Sugar: 0.4 g

# HAZELNUT TRUFFLES

*These truffles have the flavor of your favorite hazelnut spread and are just as delicious as the real thing.*

**Makes 9 fat bombs**

**2 ounces unsweetened baking chocolate**
**1 tablespoon butter**
**1 tablespoon cream cheese**
**6 tablespoons toasted hazelnuts, finely chopped, divided**
**2 tablespoons confectioners' Swerve**
**2 drops stevia glycerite**
**½ teaspoon liquid hazelnut flavor**

**1** In a small double boiler over medium-low heat, melt chocolate while slowly stirring.

**2** Add butter, cream cheese, 3 tablespoons hazelnuts, Swerve, stevia, and hazelnut flavor to chocolate and mix well until incorporated.

**3** Remove from heat and keep stirring about 10 seconds.

**4** Cool at room temperature about 1 hour until ganache has solidified.

**5** Scoop ganache with a spoon and form 9 little balls. You might want to wear plastic gloves to help keep the chocolate from sticking to your hands.

**6** Place remaining chopped hazelnuts on a medium plate and roll truffles through to coat evenly.

## Balls or Shapes?

You can use fun silicone molds to make your truffles into shapes like hearts or seashells. Just pour the ganache straight from the saucepan into the molds and then refrigerate until solid. When ready, remove from the molds and roll in coating agent.

**Per Serving**
Calories: 87 | Fat: 7.6 g | Protein: 1.7 g | Sodium: 7 mg | Fiber: 1.5 g | Carbohydrates: 5.1 g | Net Carbohydrates: 0.0 g | Sugar Alcohols: 3.3 g | Sugar: 0.3 g

# CASHEW BUTTER CUP FAT BOMBS

*Many commercially available cashew butters contain an added sweetener, so be careful when choosing one. If you can't find one at the store, you can always make your own.*

**Serves 12**

1 cup coconut oil
¾ cup unsalted butter, divided
6 tablespoons unsweetened cocoa powder
15 drops liquid stevia
¼ cup no-sugar-added unsalted cashew butter
2 tablespoons heavy whipping cream

**1** Put coconut oil, ½ cup butter, cocoa powder, and stevia in a small saucepan and stir over medium heat until melted and well combined.

**2** Pour an equal amount of the mixture into each well of a mini muffin tin lined with cupcake wrappers. Place muffin tin in the freezer and allow to harden, about 30 minutes.

**3** Place remaining ¼ cup butter, cashew butter, and whipping cream in a small bowl and beat with a handheld mixer until combined and fluffy.

**4** Once the chocolate mixture in the freezer has hardened, spoon an equal amount of the cashew butter mixture on top of each well and place in the freezer. Allow to harden, at least 30 minutes.

**5** Store in refrigerator until ready to eat.

## Nut Butters at Home

Making cashew butter is the same basic process as making coconut butter. To make about 1½ cups of cashew butter, put 2 cups unroasted, unsalted cashews in a food processor with a pinch of salt and 1 tablespoon coconut oil. Process about 30 seconds and then scrape down the sides of the food processor. Continue processing until smooth, scraping the sides when necessary.

**Per Serving**
Calories: 304 | Fat: 31.5 g | Protein: 1.6 g | Sodium: 3 mg | Fiber: 1.1 g | Carbohydrates: 3.1 g | Net Carbohydrates: 2.0 g | Sugar: 0.1 g

# SALTED CARAMEL AND BRIE BALLS

*You will love this super-easy and fast recipe. It features only three ingredients and takes less than 5 minutes to make.*

**Makes 6 fat bombs**

½ cup (4 ounces) roughly chopped Brie
¼ cup salted macadamia nuts
½ teaspoon caramel flavor

**1** In a small food processor, process all ingredients until they form a coarse dough, about 30 seconds.

**2** Form mixture into 6 balls with the aid of a spoon.

**3** Serve immediately or refrigerate up to 3 days.

**Per Serving**
Calories: 102 | Fat: 9.0 g | Protein: 4.4 g | Sodium: 119 mg | Fiber: 0.4 g | Carbohydrates: 0.8 g | Net Carbohydrates: 0.4 g | Sugar: 0.3 g

# LEMON CHEESECAKE FAT BOMBS

*Fresh lemon juice straight from the lemon is best for this recipe, but if you're out of lemons, you can use bottled versions too.*

**Serves 12**

**2 ounces (¼ cup) cream cheese, softened**
**⅔ cup unsalted butter**
**2 tablespoons heavy whipping cream**
**1 tablespoon lemon juice**
**¼ teaspoon lemon extract**
**10 drops liquid stevia**

**1** Beat cream cheese, butter, and whipping cream together in a small bowl until smooth. Add lemon juice, lemon extract, and stevia until combined.

**2** Drop by tablespoons onto a cookie sheet lined with wax paper and place in the freezer until hardened, about 30 minutes.

**3** Store in the refrigerator until ready to eat.

**Per Serving**
Calories: 115 | Fat: 11.8 g | Protein: 0.4 g | Sodium: 19 mg | Fiber: 0.0 g | Carbohydrates: 0.4 g | Net Carbohydrates: 0.4 g | Sugar: 0.3 g

# PEANUT BUTTER FAT BOMBS

*The crunchy peanut butter and crushed peanuts in this recipe give these Peanut Butter Fat Bombs an unbeatable texture. If you prefer less crunch, use smooth peanut butter instead.*

**Serves 12**

1 cup coconut oil

½ cup unsalted butter

½ cup no-sugar-added unsalted crunchy peanut butter

2 tablespoons cream cheese

10 drops liquid stevia

¼ cup crushed unsalted peanuts

**1** Place coconut oil, butter, peanut butter, cream cheese, and stevia in a small saucepan and stir over medium heat until melted.

**2** Sprinkle crushed peanuts evenly in each well of a 12-cup mini muffin pan. Pour peanut butter mixture over peanuts.

**3** Place in the freezer until hardened, about 30 minutes.

**4** Store in the refrigerator until ready to eat.

**Per Serving**
Calories: 313 | Fat: 31.6 g | Protein: 3.6 g | Sodium: 9 mg | Fiber: 1.3 g | Carbohydrates: 3.1 g | Net Carbohydrates: 1.8 g | Sugar: 0.6 g

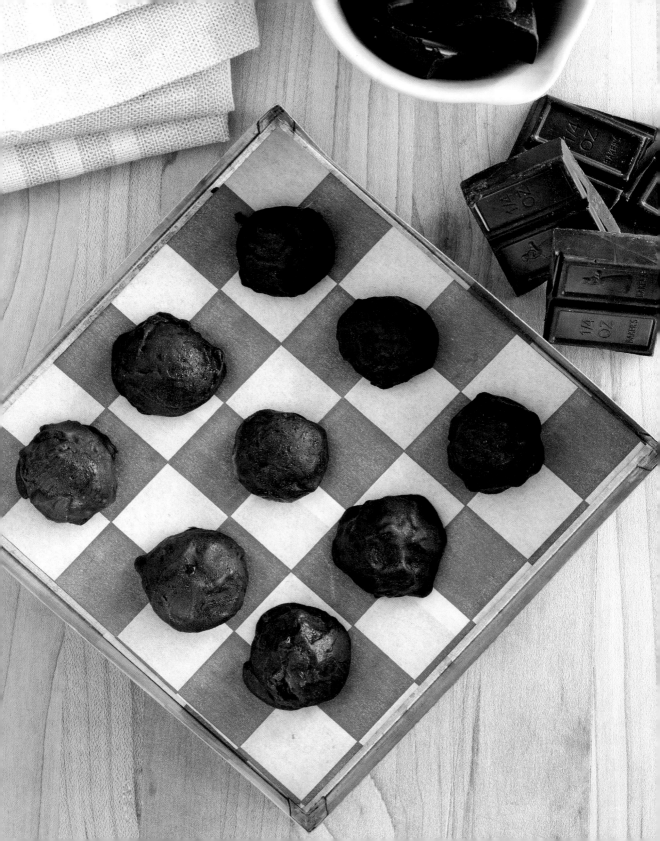

# DARK CHOCOLATE PEPPERMINT FAT BOMBS

*These fat bombs are modeled after the very famous British chocolates After Eight, which are wafer-thin dark chocolates filled with peppermint cream.*

**Makes 8 fat bombs**

**4 tablespoons coconut oil**
**4 ounces dark unsweetened baking chocolate**
**¼ teaspoon peppermint extract**
**5 drops stevia glycerite**

**1** In a small saucepan over very low heat, add coconut oil and chocolate, stirring until completely melted, about 3 minutes.

**2** Remove from heat and stir in peppermint extract and stevia.

**3** Pour into 8 silicone molds. Refrigerate until hard.

**4** Remove from molds. Serve immediately or store in refrigerator up to 1 week.

**Per Serving**
Calories: 149 | Fat: 13.5 g | Protein: 2.0 g | Sodium: 3 mg | Fiber: 2.4 g | Carbohydrates: 4.0 g | Net Carbohydrates: 1.6 g | Sugar: 0.1 g

# BLUEBERRY FAT BOMBS

*Blueberries and cream cheese are a winning combination, but if you want a different flavor, make this a triple-berry fat bomb by using a combination of blueberries, blackberries, and strawberries.*

**Serves 12**

¾ cup blueberries, divided
¼ cup unsweetened coconut cream
2½ ounces (about ⅓ cup) cream cheese, softened
½ cup coconut butter, melted
½ cup coconut oil, melted
8 drops liquid stevia

**1** Place ½ cup berries, coconut cream, and cream cheese in a food processor and process until smooth. Add coconut butter, coconut oil, and stevia and process again until smooth.

**2** Fill up each well of a 12-cup silicone mold or mini muffin tin lined with cupcake wrappers with an equal amount of the blueberry mixture and drop the remaining blueberries on top.

**3** Place in the freezer until hardened, about 30 minutes. Store in the refrigerator.

**Per Serving**
Calories: 186 | Fat: 17.9 g | Protein: 1.3 g | Sodium: 25 mg | Fiber: 1.7 g | Carbohydrates: 3.9 g | Net Carbohydrates: 2.2 g | Sugar: 1.8 g

## Use What You've Got

Silicone molds are extremely helpful when you're on a ketogenic diet, especially if you're planning to make fat bombs a regular part of your diet. If you don't want to purchase silicone molds, you can use ice cube trays, but it will be harder to remove the bombs from the trays.

# ABOUT
# THE AUTHOR

**LINDSAY BOYERS, CHNC,** is a holistic nutritionist with a background in functional nutrition and extensive experience in a wide range of dietary therapies, including the ketogenic diet. Her articles on nutrition and health have been published on various health and wellness sites, including Healthline.com, Livestrong.com, and JillianMichaels.com. She is the author of *The Everything® Guide to Gut Health, The Everything® Metabolism Diet Cookbook, The Everything® Guide to the Ketogenic Diet, The Everything® Low-Carb Meal Prep Cookbook, The Everything® Ketogenic Diet Cookbook,* and *The Everything® Guide to Intermittent Fasting.*

# US/METRIC CONVERSION CHART

## VOLUME CONVERSIONS

| US Volume Measure | Metric Equivalent |
| --- | --- |
| ⅛ teaspoon | 0.5 milliliter |
| ¼ teaspoon | 1 milliliter |
| ½ teaspoon | 2 milliliters |
| 1 teaspoon | 5 milliliters |
| ½ tablespoon | 7 milliliters |
| 1 tablespoon (3 teaspoons) | 15 milliliters |
| 2 tablespoons (1 fluid ounce) | 30 milliliters |
| ¼ cup (4 tablespoons) | 60 milliliters |
| ⅓ cup | 90 milliliters |
| ½ cup (4 fluid ounces) | 125 milliliters |
| ⅔ cup | 160 milliliters |
| ¾ cup (6 fluid ounces) | 180 milliliters |
| 1 cup (16 tablespoons) | 250 milliliters |
| 1 pint (2 cups) | 500 milliliters |
| 1 quart (4 cups) | 1 liter (about) |

*(continued on next page ▶)*

## WEIGHT CONVERSIONS

| US Weight Measure | Metric Equivalent |
| --- | --- |
| ½ ounce | 15 grams |
| 1 ounce | 30 grams |
| 2 ounces | 60 grams |
| 3 ounces | 85 grams |
| ¼ pound (4 ounces) | 115 grams |
| ½ pound (8 ounces) | 225 grams |
| ¾ pound (12 ounces) | 340 grams |
| 1 pound (16 ounces) | 454 grams |

## OVEN TEMPERATURE CONVERSIONS

| Degrees Fahrenheit | Degrees Celsius |
|---|---|
| 200 degrees F | 95 degrees C |
| 250 degrees F | 120 degrees C |
| 275 degrees F | 135 degrees C |
| 300 degrees F | 150 degrees C |
| 325 degrees F | 160 degrees C |
| 350 degrees F | 180 degrees C |
| 375 degrees F | 190 degrees C |
| 400 degrees F | 205 degrees C |
| 425 degrees F | 220 degrees C |
| 450 degrees F | 230 degrees C |

(*continued on next page* ▶)

## BAKING PAN SIZES

| American | Metric |
|---|---|
| 8 x 1½ inch round baking pan | 20 x 4 cm cake tin |
| 9 x 1½ inch round baking pan | 23 x 3.5 cm cake tin |
| 11 x 7 x 1½ inch baking pan | 28 x 18 x 4 cm baking tin |
| 13 x 9 x 2 inch baking pan | 30 x 20 x 5 cm baking tin |
| 2 quart rectangular baking dish | 30 x 20 x 3 cm baking tin |
| 15 x 10 x 2 inch baking pan | 30 x 25 x 2 cm baking tin (Swiss roll tin) |
| 9 inch pie plate | 22 x 4 or 23 x 4 cm pie plate |
| 7 or 8 inch springform pan | 18 or 20 cm springform or loose bottom cake tin |
| 9 x 5 x 3 inch loaf pan | 23 x 13 x 7 cm or 2 lb narrow loaf or pate tin |
| 1½ quart casserole | 1.5 liter casserole |
| 2 quart casserole | 2 liter casserole |

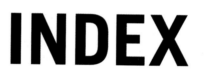

**INDEX**

# A

# B